1996

HEALTHCARE MARKETING IN TRANSITION

Practical Answers to Pressing Questions

TERRENCE J. RYNNE

A Healthcare 2000 Publication

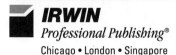

IRWIN
Professional Publishing®
Chicago • London • Singapore

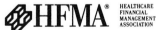 HFMA® HEALTHCARE
FINANCIAL
MANAGEMENT
ASSOCIATION

A **2000** *PUBLICATION*

ISBN 1-55738-635-8

Printed in the United States of America

BB

2 3 4 5 6 7 8 9 0

ZGraphics, Ltd.

CONTENTS

INTRODUCTION

The Healthcare Marketing Paradigm Shift

Healthcare marketing is changing fundamentally because the healthcare purchase decision—both in content and context—is changing fundamentally.

Marketing is the science and art of understanding how humans make choices, how to respond to those choices, and how to influence choices. Therefore, as the content and context of healthcare choices or purchase decisions change, what is being marketed—and where and how it is marketed—also changes.

Question: Why is the healthcare purchase decision changing?

Answer: Market forces are dictating the change.

Employers are driving the change as they try to control their ever-escalating and unpredictable healthcare benefit costs.

Employers change in three stages. By the time they reach the third stage, the healthcare purchase decision made by their employees will be fundamentally different, and healthcare marketing will be working under a new paradigm: a radically changed framework for understanding and handling the new business situation.

The three steps of employer change are:

1) Employers become concerned about rising healthcare benefits/ costs, figure out what their options are, and determine to begin exerting their influence on the market. Employer coalitions or single large employers in a given market decide to use their muscle—

their power to steer employees to one set of healthcare providers or another.

2) Employers insist on, and get, preferred, lower rates from physicians and hospitals in exchange for offering their employees a benefit package that includes—or even steers employees to—those preferred providers. The steering mechanism is financial incentives in the form of lower out-of-pocket costs to the employees for using the preferred providers, and higher out-of-pocket expenditures if they choose out-of-network providers. This occurs either through direct contracts or through a PPO, preferred provider organization.

Lower rates satisfy employers for a time if their overall benefit costs go down or the rate of increase moderates significantly, and if they then can predict in their own financial planning what this key variable in their cost structures will be from year to year.

Unfortunately for employers, however, their overall healthcare benefit costs are not just a function of unit costs, they are also a function of the number of units. In a PPO arrangement, there may be an acceptable rate per unit, but typically there aren't sufficient controls on utilization. Healthcare benefit costs will not decrease if utilization of services increases, despite a hard-won, toughly negotiated lower rate. Moreover, without such controls on utilization, employers can't predict with any assurance what their costs will be from year to year.

3) Enter the capitation option. (*Capus* is Latin for head. *Capitation* means fixed payment per head.)

If employers pay a fixed fee per employee each year to a set of healthcare providers to handle all their employees' healthcare, it is up to those providers to find ways to manage that care without losing money. All the incentives change. Instead of providers receiving more money for every unit of service—whether it is truly required or not—units of service *cost* providers.

Employers in a capitated arrangement are able to predict their healthcare benefit costs and shift the financial risk of handling very expensive cases to the providers.

Question: How does one know when the change will hit a given market? How does one know how quickly the change will proceed? How can one gauge how quickly the market might shift away from the old paradigm to the new paradigm?

Answer: There are eight indicators that allow a healthcare marketer to gauge how quickly a market will reach a tipping point.

Each of these indicators is weighted in points, and an individual market is scored in terms of its readiness for capitation, i.e., how quickly it will shift to an HMO option if an attractive option is presented.

Those indicators for gauging how quickly employers will jump into capitation are as follows:

1) Is a percentage of the employer community self-insured?

+ 3 points

Self-insured employers carry all the risk. Therefore, if their employee healthcare costs are on the rise, self-insured employers will—all things being equal—have a very direct interest in moderating the increases or reducing costs. They will be even more interested than those whose health insurance premiums are on the rise but who share that risk with health insurers and/or health providers.

2) Has a large percentage of employers closely studied the issues involved in controlling healthcare costs?

+ 2 points

In some markets, benefits managers and chief executives are not truly that focused on their healthcare premiums and healthcare costs. Either they have not had a problem big enough to command their undivided attention, or they are so concentrated on other strategic problems or opportunities, that they have not yet made it an important item on their management agenda.

In other markets, key executives have become very concerned, conversant, and involved. There's plenty of lip service, with "sky-rocketing-healthcare-costs" being used as one word all across the country. However, the amount of actual, intelligent concern and behavior varies greatly across the country. Typically, if there is concern, immersion in the issues, and an understanding of what companies in other markets around the country have done to control healthcare costs, there will soon be action.

3) Do employers have financial difficulties of their own?

+ 3 points

To the degree that companies are aggressively looking for ways to cut costs or increase margins, they will probably be looking at healthcare insurance premiums or healthcare costs as an area in which to save money. On the other hand, if they are doing well financially and their cost structures are not perceived as problematic, they will focus less aggressively on healthcare costs.

It surprised everyone, for example, that in the recently completed round of labor negotiations with the United Auto Workers, the Big Three auto companies did not negotiate more aggressively on healthcare benefits. The healthcare benefit package is still quite rich and allows for a significant amount of choice. After all, in recent years, even the public has heard the canards about health insurance outstripping steel in the auto manufacturers' cost structures. But with the increased number of autos sold, increasing profits, and a large volume of units over which to spread costs, the Big three were not very aggressive in the recent round of negotiations, either on reducing the size of the healthcare benefit package or on reducing the amount of choice workers currently enjoy. Other employers in the Detroit area are following these bellwether employers.

4) Have employers become disenchanted with "discount medicine"?

+ 5 points

Employers have worked with PPOs and enjoyed some short-term reductions, but over time, their premiums again began to rise. The unit cost of a given unit of service may have been less, but that didn't mean overall costs went down because there were no controls on *utilization*. They can't, therefore, predict their healthcare costs for a given year.

As a result, they are ready for an approach that shares risk with them, that gives them a fixed price for the year, and that has built-in mechanisms for controlling utilization, i.e., a capitated HMO.

5) Are employers already involved in contracts that in effect "steer" employees to one provider over another?

+ 4 points

When employers have begun to work with their employees to have them choose a more limited panel of providers, they have begun to be aware of, anticipate, and handle employee misgivings and questions. They relish good, credible information on quality and price so they can keep their employees supplied with information that eases employees' misgivings.

6) Are there healthcare competitors in the marketplace ready with a comprehensive capitated product?

+ 2–5 points

If a competitor is ready with an appropriate, comprehensive package of physicians, hospitals, and other services at a capitated rate, employers—depending on their trust in and regard for that entity and the degree of employee resistance they anticipate to that entity—may go for the package very quickly.

7) Are there organized discussions between employers over health-care issues, i.e., "Is there an employer coalition forming"?

+ 3 points

If employers are communicating with one another, they are more likely to answer misgivings that may arise, find solutions to stumbling blocks, and find ways to make capitation come sooner than if they remained in isolation.

8) Is there a gadfly/energizer/leader in the employer community?

+ 2 points

The process is hastened if one or more employers get the bit between their teeth and actively prepare the way for others.

Two additional questions for predicting how a marketplace will play out over time:

- How important to employers are their employee benefit plans as management tools?

- How closely do they listen to their employees' wants and preferences when it comes to healthcare providers?

Legend: 24 to 27 points: It's upon you.

20 to 23 points: It's imminent.

16 to 19 points: It's coming.

Under 16 points: Relax for the moment—
but keep checking.

HEALTHCARE MARKETING UNDER A NEW PARADIGM

Healthcare marketing is shifting from one paradigm to another. From day to day, healthcare marketers are living between the times. In fact, many are living under all three eras at once: the old, the between, and the new. That can make life very challenging to say the least. Depending on the marketplace, we will have to be practicing partly under the old paradigm of healthcare decision making; working out of the old in transition to the new; and at the same time, planning for and sometimes practicing as if we are already in the new era.

Understanding the demands of each paradigm and understanding when to shift from one to the other will be key for our psychological and professional survival. All of us like simplicity. We prefer to be in one place or another, rather than in three places simultaneously. Unfortunately, for many markets across the country, we are living in all three worlds, under all three paradigms at once. Therefore, it will be awhile before we are able to move lock, stock, and barrel from the old paradigm into the new.

The change in the healthcare purchase decision/paradigm will influence the way healthcare marketers relate to their four important constituents: **physicians, consumers, employers,** and **managed-care providers.** We'll take each constituency, one at a time, and explore how healthcare marketing changes from the old to the new through the between.

What Is the Old Paradigm?

In the old paradigm, consumers choose physicians; physicians choose hospitals; and insurance programs pick up the tab—either insurance programs provided through employers, or insurance programs provided through the government—namely Medicare, Medicaid, and CHAMPUS.

What Is the New Paradigm?

In the new paradigm, the purchase decision is made by employees at the time their employers offer them alternative insurance and provider arrangements. Employees choose their physicians, their hospitals, and their other healthcare providers at the same moment as they choose their insurance. It is all bundled together in one package.

Under the old paradigm, healthcare marketers marketed physicians and hospitals to employers, consumers, and managed-care companies. In the new paradigm, the healthcare marketer markets an entire package of health services and insurance—first to the employer in order to be placed in front of the consumer, and then to the consumer, i.e., the employee, who makes the final purchase decision. That change, as simple as it sounds, changes almost all that the healthcare marketer does and focuses on from day to day.

We'll trace how the shift in the healthcare purchase decision paradigm changes marketing. We'll also trace what life is like in the no-man's land between the paradigms.

Our main thesis is that many healthcare marketers will need to be doing activities appropriate to all three paradigms at once, because they will be existing in all three worlds at once. From day to day, they will be doing activities that match the old paradigm, that match reality in the era between the paradigms, and that are appropriate for taking advantage of the new paradigm.

Does this mean that healthcare marketers should stop doing what they are doing? Is all that they have learned to do out of date?

The key for healthcare marketers is to know the *timing* of when to shift resources from old, to between, to new paradigm activities, as well as to know the *mix* of old, between, and new paradigm activities required by a particular market.

For example, if a market is still heavily fee-for-service, all the old paradigm activities still make complete sense. In many markets, hospitals are only now taking full advantage of the pull of some of their key service lines.

In addition, very few markets are heavily capitated. Even in heavily capitated markets, old paradigm activities still have some relevance.

Finally, some activities are effective across all three paradigms—such as good market research, public relations, and focusing on women and newcomers. Even image advertising is making a comeback, but now it is to build brand equity for the Integrated Health System instead of for the hospital.

CHAPTER 1

Healthcare Marketing: What to Do Between the Times

Figures 1-1 through 1-4 are overview grids that depict the activities under each of the three paradigms, as well as how healthcare marketing changes—depending on the status of a given market's evolution.

The figures present the differences between healthcare marketing under the old and new paradigms of healthcare decision making, as well as what is different about the era "between the times"—i.e., while the old makes its way to, and overlaps with, the new.

Activities are shown according to the four customer constituents of healthcare marketing.

Figure 1-1: Marketing to Consumers

Old Paradigm	Between the Times	New Paradigm
Position the hospital	Build a true system	Position the system
Community relations	Community benefit	Community health status improvement
Wellness as gift to community and loss leader	Wellness as strategy for bonding with employers	Wellness as serious business contributing to financial success
Hospital service line marketing	Hospital service line direct contracting and marketing	System-wide service line management and marketing
Attract fee-for-service business	Build a book of managed-care business • Focus on the Medicare business • Develop managed-care capability for Medicaid business	Capture X00,000 covered lives • Convert Medicare business to Medicare risk contracting • Capitated Medicaid business
Inbound telemarketing	Inbound and outbound telemarketing	Communications center
Advertising and public relations: service lines	Advertising and public relations: hospital branding	Advertising and public relations: system branding

Figure 1-2: Marketing to Physicians

Old Paradigm	Between the Times	New Paradigm
Cater to specialists	Negotiate with specialists	Retrain specialists
Help MDs attract more fee-for-service business	Help MDs attract and hang on to managed-care business	Help MDs handle a panel of patients
Satisfy primary-care physicians	Acquire primary-care physician practices	Free primary-care MDs from headaches that distract from patient care
Information to MDs on their financial performance vis-à-vis the hospital	Information to MDs on their clinical performance vis-à-vis peers	Information to MDs on their financial and clinical performance vis-à-vis benchmark performers

Figure 1-3: Marketing to Employers

Old Paradigm	Between the Times	New Paradigm
Networking	Carve out contracts	Full capitation
Build relations	Provide models of cost containment	Partner in benefit design

Figure 1-4: Marketing to PPOs and HMOs

Old Paradigm	Between the Times	New Paradigm
The more relationships the merrier	Choose partners	Dance close
Stand-alone marketing	Stand-apart marketing	Co-marketing

CONSUMER MARKETING UNDER THE OLD PARADIGM

Old Paradigm	Between the Times	New Paradigm
Position the hospital	Build a true system	Position the system

Old Paradigm: Position the Hospital

Under the old paradigm, the challenge for the healthcare marketer is to position the hospital in the mind of consumers in such a way that they are positive about the hospital, drawn to it, and will even push physicians to select that hospital when they need hospitalization.

Brand equity is definitely in the hospital. When the marketplace thinks health, it thinks physicians and hospitals. The challenge for the marketer is to differentiate one brand of hospital from another through the many methods of effective positioning and communications. (See Chapter 5 for a step-by-step guide to enhancing the brand equity of a healthcare organization.)

Between the Times: Build a True System

In the era between the times, the healthcare marketer is doing everything possible to enhance the brand image of the hospital, recognizing that the reputation of the hospital or hospitals within an integrated healthcare delivery system will be one key criterion that customers use when choosing their packages at enrollment time every year. But clearly, the healthcare marketer is aware that at a certain time, resources need to be shifted from the image enhancement of the hospital to making the entire *system* a household word in the mind of the consumer.

Question: When does one stop marketing the hospital and begin marketing and positioning the integrated healthcare delivery system?

Answer: When the marketplace's employers reach a 30-percent level in terms of capitation, it is time to begin shifting to the new paradigm.

New Paradigm: Position the System

In the new paradigm, the challenge for the healthcare marketer is to position the integrated healthcare delivery system by clarifying the meaning of the product category and enhancing the image of the particular brand. Consumers choose one integrated healthcare delivery system/insurance package or another when they make their healthcare purchase decision. In the new paradigm, therefore, the healthcare marketer at a certain point stops marketing the hospital and transitions to marketing the system.

Old Paradigm	Between the Times	New Paradigm
Community relations	Community benefit	Community health status improvement

Old Paradigm: Community Relations

An important part of consumer-oriented healthcare marketing has always been community relations: outreach, programming, and networking.

A hospital is an important community resource, dependent for its success upon the positive goodwill and support of the community. Enlightened marketers invest significant energy and resources into community outreach and networking. By involving significant numbers of people in the affairs of a hospital, they bring those people up close and give them a day-to-day active interest in the affairs of the hospital. As a "low interest" category, healthcare is not a product that people purchase frequently. By keeping the issues and concerns of a hospital in front of the community in an ongoing way, people are more likely to think of that hospital when they need healthcare.

Moreover, by involving networks of positive word-of-mouth supporters, the main messages hospital leadership wants to get out to the community can be conveyed quickly and efficiently.

A further aim of good community relations is to have the community make the hospital a focus of its concern and fund-raising.

Hospitals that neglect community relations suffer the consequences. Those that enjoy the strongest and deepest support from the community compete most successfully.

Between the Times: Community Benefit

Between the times, a hospital does less telling the community about itself and does more listening to the community about its needs. Many hospitals pass through a time of community suspicion. During this time, not-for-profit hospitals need to prove themselves deserving of not-for-profit status. For-profit hospitals have to prove that they aren't money machines and that they are still beneficent institutions deserving the community's trust and support. This leads to a time of more aggressive "community benefit" programming.

The underlying reason why political bodies such as state legislatures, county boards, and attorneys general feel free to go after hospitals' tax-exempt status is that the voters have lost the sense that hospitals have community benefit as their *raison d'etre*. When asked if hospitals are for-profit or not-for-profit, an overwhelming majority of the American public answers "for-profit." For an individual hospital to establish a clear, unassailable profile as a generous, beneficent community resource is the best protection against taxing bodies looking for new sources of income. If the general public is clear that a hospital provides extensive services for the poor and disadvantaged, is community benefit-oriented and not self serving, and provides services to the community that the government would have to provide if the hospital wasn't there, the general public will recognize that the hospital deserves tax-exempt status and will keep its elected representatives from tampering with that designation.

Calculations of the Return on Investment (ROI) of investments aimed at establishing this reputation with the community and preserving tax-exempt status are straightforward. Resources invested in communicating how much charity care a hospital provides; that a hospital provides programs for no other reason than community need (i.e., not to generate any financial gain); and that a hospital provides new initiatives and programs for the poor or underserved have great indirect financial return. Tax-exempt status equates to substantial real estate and corporate income tax exemptions as well as access to capital at substantially lower rates.

Consequently, the marketing function, in the period between the times, develops two separate ledgers of success and two separate budgets, one for community benefit and one for business development.

The business development objectives are stated in measurable financial terms, such as "To secure X increase in business for the cardiac services worth $X00,000 in incremental revenue."

The community benefit objectives are not any less measurable but only indirectly financial—e.g., "To secure X increase in the percentage of the target market rating the hospital a community service leader."

Marketing proceeds with both ledgers and budgets with the same management rigor: setting objectives, determining the steps most likely to achieve the objectives, and implementing and tracking progress.

New Paradigm: Community Health Status Improvement

Under the new paradigm, the community is an even more serious focus of attention. In order for a healthcare system to survive financially, it is important over time that consumers take more responsibility for their own health. The most efficient way to keep people out of hospitals and, therefore, to save resources and have something left over at the end of the year from a capitated grant, is to have people stay healthy. Poor lifestyles contribute to morbidity and mortality. For example, it is estimated that 85 percent of strokes could be prevented if people did not smoke, lost weight, exercised, didn't drink to excess, handled their stress and life problems more capably, etc. The risk factors of stroke are mainly lifestyle related.

Hospitals therefore begin to measure their success in a different way—by gauging the degree of community improvement in health status indicators. Hospitals work collaboratively with other community agencies and providers of services to influence those health gains.

Moreover, a hospital's strategic planning changes from an inside/out approach—i.e., setting priorities based on the needs of the institution—to an outside/in approach—stating priorities of the institution in terms of community health needs.

Old Paradigm	Between the Times	New Paradigm
Wellness as a gift to the community and loss leader	Wellness as a strategy for nurturing relations with employers and the business community	Wellness as serious business and behavior modification

Old Paradigm: Wellness as a Gift and Loss Leader

In the late 1970s, many hospitals across the county were caught up in the wellness movement. They recognized that even though their stated mission was "health" care, they really only provided "sickness" care. They began to broaden their operative definition of health care and began to offer more health education, screening, and health promotion services to the community.

This was also the era of business diversification. Hospitals formed multiple corporations and made multiple attempts to get into other business lines than just the hospital business. There was some sense that there was money to be made in wellness. Very soon, however, hospitals realized that there wasn't much money to be made from the mainline health promotion and wellness services—unless they went full blown into a fitness center facility and program mode. Gradually they began to see that health promotion and wellness services were loss leader services. When hospitals continued to offer them they offered them as gifts to the community, less out of business diversification motives and more clearly out of their civic responsibility for the community's overall health and well-being.

Between the Times: Wellness as a Strategy with Employers

The one part of the overall health promotion service umbrella that proved to be profitable was the industrial wellness part of the service. When hospitals tuned in to helping employers reduce their workers' compensation costs, they found a way to not only serve the employer but generate profits.

As the relationship with area employers became even more important to monitor and manage, these services became not just a way to generate revenue, but also a way to demonstrate effectively to employers that a given hospital was not only concerned about helping them reduce their overall healthcare cost—they also were competent in doing so.

One hospital in Southern Wisconsin, for example, established industrial health centers close to clusters of small- and mid-size manufacturing companies. At the centers they offered appropriate employee health physicals, urgent care for injured workers, appropriate diagnostic testing for meeting OSHA requirements, and effective case management services.

Over time, the industrial services became so successful that they were able to target employers with large workers' compensation costs and offer to provide services free—only asking that they be given one half of the *savings* the employer would experience on its workers' compensation bill. Through effective on-site industrial nursing and case management and by tightening up the relationships with the emergency department and other key specialists, they were able to cut lost work time so significantly that they generated hundreds of thousands of dollars in income for the hospital from savings produced for the employers.

These services served to build very positive relationships between the sponsoring hospital and the area employers and is an effective "between the times tactic" on the way to more comprehensive contracting and capitated arrangements.

New Paradigm: Wellness as Serious Business

In a capitated environment, wellness and health behavior modification becomes a serious challenge and serious business. Wrestling with the challenge of how to help people change their lifestyles and stay healthy becomes a central business challenge, not just a peripheral pursuit.

If, for example, an integrated healthcare delivery system can persuade one of its members/clients who may be at risk for a high-risk pregnancy to comply with the dictates of good prenatal care and prevent just one premature birth, it can produce huge savings. One, $1 million, neonatal, intensive-care baby avoided will mean a rather direct savings to the organization's bottom line.

In addition, reducing the incidence of stroke or heart attack in health plan members through changed lifestyle will also be immediately financially rewarding to the organization. Working with the community to lower the teenage pregnancy rate will reduce society's healthcare bill. And finally, improving the ways that diabetic patients comply with their care will prevent unnecessary office visits and even hospitalizations. Over a whole panel of such patients, those reductions will result in the need for fewer nurses, fewer physicians, and less resources consumed in caring for the patient. As a result, the capitated contract becomes that much more lucrative for the organization.

Old Paradigm	Between the Times	New Paradigm
Hospital product line marketing	Hospital product line marketing and direct contracting	System-wide product line marketing

Old Paradigm: Hospital Product Line Marketing

In recent years, as hospital leaders began to understand that a hospital is really a bundle of businesses, leaders recognized the need to break that bundle into its major business lines. CEOs saw that they could only have a flourishing hospital if the individual business lines flourished. The maternity service, the emergency department, the cancer care service, the orthopedics service, the heart care service, were really what customers with distinct needs and problems were seeking. While the umbrella image of the hospital helped draw people to those services, the way the business actually worked was vis-à-vis these distinct customer groups in the market. Customers in need of an emergency service used different decision variables and criteria for selecting an emergency service than customers looking for an obstetrics service. This is the fundamental business reason for the development of strong service line management: to match and manage services with distinct pockets of consumer need and demand. (See Chapter 6: "Service Line Management, Marketing, and Managed Care.")

Service line management puts the right kind of executive talent and resources—when done appropriately—where they can make the most difference. The traditional organizational structure of the hospital needs to be adjusted, in some cases radically, in order for the business to be run in the way the marketplace demands. With a concentrated focus on "centers of excellence," a hospital can much more effectively leverage its marketing talent and resources.

Hospitals move away from simple-minded image campaigns and develop more and more sophisticated marketing plans and campaigns behind key clinical services. As a result, hospitals, through a combination of deft physician and consumer marketing, are able to build specific clinical services and take market share away from competitors.

The service lines are more powerful in terms of marketing if hospitals put in place the following features of a "center of excellence." Without these attributes, they are a "center" in name only. The more of these attributes, the stronger the center of excellence.

- A committed *group of collaborative specialist physicians* with excellent reputations.

  Much greater brand equity can be built with a clear single identity than can be built through the individual reputations of single practices.

- *A clear, single identity and physical location.*

  For example, Catherine McAuley Health System in Ann Arbor, Michigan, working with its cardiologists and the cardiac surgeons, established the "Michigan Heart Institute." With this name and impressive facility and program, they claimed and staked out a leadership position.

- *A single access point that makes inquiries from referring physicians simple and efficient.*

  Butterworth Hospital in Grand Rapids, Michigan, a major referral center for the western part of the State of Michigan, realized that a call from a referring physician wanting to send a patient touched off an internal sequence of seven calls to various constituents: to the residency program, to the emergency department, to housekeeping, to nursing, to admitting, etc., before the referring physician could be given a go-ahead to refer his or her patients. They realized that referring physicians were frustrated and beginning to shift business. They instituted a "one-call-does-it-all" system internally, and made the response to the inquiring referring physician immediate.

- *Coordinated, consistent approaches to patient education.*

  A strong service line comes to a consensus on a rich package of patient education done in a timely, appropriate manner—at times by physicians, at times by nurses. The approach to patient education is translated into a consistent protocol and is supported by first-rate teaching materials.

• *Nurses as patient guides.*

When nurse practitioners, clinical nurse specialists, or other nurses are involved at the entrance into the service, they establish themselves as guides for patients and serve as a glue for the program, making sure that communications are centered on the patient and that patients are fully informed at each step of the care continuum.

The Center for Breast Health, for example, at Mt. Sinai Health System in Cleveland, has two key nurses who work hand-in-hand with the physicians and serve as the guides and patient advocates through the entire experience of recovering from breast cancer. They don't supplant the physicians' role in caring and communication. They enhance it. In fact, they make the life of the physicians that much more productive and efficient.

• *Information systems* are put in place that allow service line leadership and staff to track *financial, clinical, and marketing performance.*

As a result, physicians have the ability to relate clinical practice outcomes with financial objectives and see their relationships. Such data serve as the basis for clinical pathway development and for developing true package pricing.

• *Outreach to other professionals.*

For example, Tallahassee Memorial Regional Medical Center built a Heart Institute with well-equipped rooms for resident education, continuing medical education, and ongoing programs for nurses working in the cardiology field. Such courses established Tallahassee Memorial Regional Medical Center as a preeminent provider of services and built strong interactive relationships with physicians and nurses in the region.

Between the Times: Hospital Product Line Direct Contracting

With these key components of an authentic "center of excellence," or service line, hospitals are in a position to respond to the opportunity in the market for carving out direct contracting. Everything hospitals have done under the old paradigm prepares them for success "between the times." Because they have physicians working together; have established the information they need to develop a convincing story to area industries on both cost and quality; and are able to develop a true package price because they know their fixed and incremental costs for providing a service, they are able to successfully negotiate direct contracts for key clinical services.

New Paradigm: System-Wide Product Lines

As the employer moves away from discounted contractual arrangements for services, looks for stronger utilization controls, and desires to share risk with providers, the service line management structure begins to change as well. No longer is it an individual hospital contracting with employers. It is now a comprehensive system of physicians, hospitals, and other healthcare providers entering into comprehensive capitated contracts.

As physicians' and hospitals' financial incentives are more aligned and as the hospitals and doctors see the value of working closely together to provide an excellent clinical service at the lowest possible cost, it becomes apparent that, for a given region, a hospital-based approach to service line management should give way to a system-wide approach.

Instead of doing multiple marketing plans, a system does one. Instead of developing multiple, individual chest-pain programs and campaigns, systems do one coordinated approach and campaign. Such an approach requires that, over time, the physicians begin to identify more with the system as their partner than with any individual hospital. That has immediate implications for capital investment, technology, and relations between the facilities. It also means the end of the medical arms race between facilities in the same system.

As the system identity of the key clinical services strengthens in the mind of the market, the overall identity of the system and its drawing power begins to strengthen. If the system has a reputation for providing first-rate specialized clinical services, it is a more attractive contracting partner for managed care. A multi-hospital system is more appropriate as a contracting partner for employers that have an employee base in many geographic locations.

Franciscan Health System in Aston, Pennsylvania, for example, has been working for the last few years to change its key clinical services from hospital-based service lines to system-wide service lines. They are doing that to assure the same high level of quality across all the facilities within the system; to use resources more efficiently and effectively; and to build an identity in the marketplace that unites and transcends the identities of the individual hospitals in the system.

Old Paradigm	Between the Times	New Paradigm
Attract fee-for-service business	Build a managed-care book of business	Capture X00,000 covered lives

Old Paradigm: Attract Fee-for-Service

The focus of many marketing programs in recent years has been on the fee-for-service, indemnity market. By attracting such patients, hospitals are able to offset their contractual adjustments from other types of patients, in particular, Medicare and Medicaid patients.

Payor mix in the old paradigm is a key number to watch and manage.

Between the Times: Build Managed Care

As a marketplace shifts away from indemnity insurance, it becomes very important for the hospital to learn how to manage the managed-care base of its business effectively. In a managed-care environment, whole blocks of business can be lost through managed-care contracts. Without a critical mass of patients, a hospital can't survive for very long. The hospital then focuses on building an adequate book of managed-care business.

In this situation, one important group is still left—however, with individual free choice—and that is Medicare patients. In effect, Medicare patients are still acting under the old paradigm. They choose the physicians, and the physicians choose the hospital. Insurance—in this case, the government—picks up the bill.

In this between the times era, therefore, Medicare patients re-emerge as an attractive target market. As hospitals are learning to handle their costs more appropriately, and survive with managed-care business, they find themselves better able to operate profitably with Medicare reimbursement. Senior membership programs make a comeback.

One major Midwest system, for example, finds that reimbursement from Medicare is greater than what it is receiving from its own HMO.

Medicaid patients, too, still have a degree of free choice and are, in effect, operating under the old paradigm. Every indication, however, points to the need for states to develop managed care, if not capitated contracts, for Medicaid patients. They recognize what employers have recognized before them. Hospitals begin to put together the systems and the networks that can handle managed-care Medicaid contracts.

New Paradigm: Capture Covered Lives

As a market shifts to capitated contracts, it is then important for the integrated healthcare delivery system to capture an adequate number of covered lives to make it viable for all the parties concerned. In the Chicago area, for example, every burgeoning integrated healthcare delivery system has a similar key goal with almost exactly the same targets. Northwestern, Rush-Presbyterian-St. Luke's, and the University of Chicago, for example, all indicate that they are aiming to have X-million covered lives in their system within a few years. The competitive lines are drawn.

In the new paradigm, the Medicare business also begins to change. In many markets, especially in the South and West, managed-care companies have made Medicare patients a marketing target and are enrolling them in Medicare risk contracts. In effect, these contracts are capitated arrangements in which the healthcare delivery partners and the insurance partner share a capitated fee for each enrolled person. It is up to the partners, then, to provide total care for the over-65 patient, for a fixed amount of money. By aligning the financial incentives between physicians and hospitals, many provider participants in these programs have found them to be very profitable. In the new paradigm, therefore, even the Medicare patient shifts out of an old paradigm framework and moves into the new paradigm. Finally, systems working effectively in a managed-care environment find that they can handle X-thousands of Medicaid covered lives effectively—as long as the capitated payment is appropriate.

Old Paradigm	Between the Times	New Paradigm
Inbound telemarketing	Outbound telemarketing	A communications center

Old Paradigm: Inbound Telemarketing

With a focus on fee-for-service patients, a hospital's physician-referral service is a very powerful lever for generating business. A certain percentage of a given marketplace is at any one time looking for a physician, either because they are new to a market, are finally admitting that they are not immortal, or have been dissatisfied with a previous physician. A certain portion of those people find a hospital to be a credible, central source for physician recommendations. An aggressive physician-referral program is therefore a basic tool for strengthening relations with a private medical staff and eventually for generating additional business for the hospital.

Effective physician-referral programs include aggressive marketing campaigns and sophisticated, well-trained staff to hear and respond to community requests, to make sure that the appointment for the patient is made, and that the whole experience is smooth and easy for the patient as well as for the medical staff. Moreover, physician-referral services have evolved to the point where they can track, over time, a patient that enters their system through the physician referral service, and therefore, establish and clearly demonstrate the return that the investment in the overall physician referral service secures.

Between the Times: Outbound Telemarketing

This inbound telemarketing capability evolves into a two-way capability as hospitals recognize the cross-selling potential of effective database marketing, and make their programs ever more efficient and cost effective.

The same staff members who are responding to inquiries can also reach out to key parts of the market. A number of hospitals, for example, have established very successful newcomer programs, coupling principles of direct mail with follow-up outbound telemarketing. By definition, newcomers are looking. It makes sense to reach them first and either preempt or reinforce their neighbors' advice concerning preferred healthcare providers. One can reach them by phone before the Welcome

Wagon arrives. The same staff members who receive physician-referral inquiries reach out via the phone to newcomers.

Moreover, physician-referral programs staffed by nurses offer an even greater incentive to the market for getting in touch with the service. The availability of nurses signals not only that the physician referral will be handled by a professional, but also that a knowledgeable person is available to answer basic questions about healthcare. The "order taking" service becomes a triage service.

Just as physicians' offices have handled the double, almost contra-dictory demands of their two types of patients, namely fee-for-service and capitated, so also a hospital begins to experience the same pulls. A triage function is able to encourage some patients to come in for care while discouraging others. The triage function enables the hospital and its associated physicians to handle managed-care business more efficiently.

New Paradigm: Communications Center

The critical mass of skills and technology established through the database marketing system evolves very readily into a much more comprehensive communications center for helping to handle capitated contracts. The phone becomes an important tool for helping patients resolve problems, increase compliance levels, and maintain good health habits.

Old Paradigm	Between the Times	New Paradigm
Advertising and public relations focuses on service lines	Advertising and public relations builds hospital brand equity	Advertising and public relations builds system brand equity

Old Paradigm: Campaigns for Service Lines

Advertising and public relations that goes beyond making a splash or managing image, but truly supports the development of business and additional volume for a hospital, does so by concentrating on key ser-vice lines. The larger the self-referral quotient for a service, the more direct the relationship between advertising and public relations and additional business. Services such as the emergency service, behavioral health services, and maternity services that have a high self-referral quotient are very efficiently grown through marketing communications. Other services that have a higher physician-referral quotient can also be assisted, although less directly, by marketing communications. If a hospital's reputation for cancer care, for example, is so strong in the mind of the general populace, when physicians are contemplating a referral to a particular hospital, they can be influenced by patients with a pre-existing preference for one hospital over another.

Much of effective healthcare advertising and public relations, therefore, in recent years has been service-line oriented. Comparatively little has been aimed at building brand equity—except indirectly through the reputation of specific clinical services.

Between the Times: Hospital Positioning Campaigns

Advertising and public relations in the era between the times still has plenty of room for growing individual service lines. But it is also important to prepare for the shift in the paradigm. The overall reputation of a hospital within an integrated healthcare delivery system will be one of the key variables that helps the market choose one system over another. The Barnes/Jewish/Christian System in St. Louis, for example, benefits very much from the overall reputation of the Barnes Hospital in the marketplace.

Many burgeoning healthcare systems then adopt what in effect is a two-stage strategy. While there is still time—i.e., before the integrated healthcare delivery system is the object of the purchase decision—it makes sense to build the brand equity of the hospital. That will serve well in the short term, in the era between the times. It will also serve well to facilitate the parts of the market that are still under the old paradigm—i.e., the remnants of the indemnity market, the Medicare market, and Medicaid before managed-care contracts. Finally, it will have residual value as the system moves into the new paradigm.

New Paradigm: System Positioning Campaigns

At a certain point, it makes sense to stop putting resources into marketing the hospital and to devote energy and resources to making the system a household name. The system is what the market will be purchasing. The reputations of the individual operating units within the system, of course, will contribute to the brand equity of the system. Unless the existing brand equities, however, are tapped—i.e., linked in the public's mind with the overall system—the system will not benefit from those pre-existing reputations. The Barnes/Jewish/Christian union, for example, is named BJC, which unfortunately subordinates the name Barnes and makes the system one more example of healthcare alphabet soup.

Most systems across the country, therefore, are already changing the names of their hospitals within a system to make the link with the sponsoring organization much clearer—e.g., Fairfax Hospital, part of the INOVA system, is now clearly featuring the name of the system in all its signage and communications. The system name becomes the marquee name, while the name of the individual operating unit is featured to the degree that it can lend credibility to the system—otherwise, it is subordinated.

MARKETING TO PHYSICIANS

Old Paradigm	Between the Times	New Paradigm
Cater to specialists	Negotiate with specialists	Retrain specialists

Old Paradigm: Cater to Specialists

Until recently, hospital leaders viewed their specialists as their money-making physicians. The specialists who were well established could ask for, if not demand, significant capital expenditures in an ongoing way from a hospital board because the board of directors reviewed financial statements that indicated that those specialists were generating significant revenue for the hospital. Surgical specialists in particular generated not only hefty incomes for themselves but, according to the way the financial statements of the hospital were drawn up, were attributed significant revenue generation for the hospital.

Savvy hospital administrators and boards always knew, of course, that the real source of the hospital's financial performance was the primary-care physician, but from day to day, as specialists perform surgery, take referrals into specialized units, perform specialized testing, and reimbursement from insurance companies comes into the hospital under their names, they—not the primary-care physicians—seemed to be the key to a hospital's success.

Well-known specialists were the plums of recruitment efforts. They helped the hospital project a quality image to the marketplace. The hospital was perceived as an up-to-date mecca for healing to the degree that it had on its staff specialists who were well-trained.

Between the Times: Negotiate with Specialists

As hospitals participate in managed-care plans, the primary-care physicians come to the fore. Primary-care physicians are prized if they use resources appropriately and if they do not make unnecessary referrals to specialists. To the degree that primary-care physicians practice with efficiency, the fewer the resources consumed by a healthcare system.

Managed-care providers rate and rank primary-care physicians. They pursue for their panels those that practice quality medicine efficiently.

As hospitals come together with their physicians to form physician hospital organizations with an eye towards comprehensive contracts, primary-care physicians come to the fore. Just as they are key for managed-care companies, they are key for comprehensive, capitated contracts. As hospitals and physicians develop PHOs, the leadership mantle falls to the primary-care physicians. It is up to them to determine through negotiations with specialists what percent of the healthcare dollar goes to specialists and what percent of the healthcare dollar stays with them. Specialists, more clearly than ever, recognize how business flows to them or doesn't flow to them.

New Paradigm: Retrain Specialists

The proportion of specialists to primary-care physicians in capitated situations is typically way out of balance. The number of specialist physicians usually far outstrips the number of primary-care physicians. Hospital after hospital, integrated healthcare system after integrated healthcare system, recognizes the need to redress the proportion.

Stanford University Hospital, for example, recently reported proudly that it had recruited 45 of the 100 primary-care physicians it was planning to recruit. Every university hospital in the country seems to have the same goal at the same time. Everyone is simultaneously looking for 100 or more additional primary-care physicians.

Concomitantly, the realization dawns that perhaps there are enough physicians, just too many specialists. Many specialists begin to accept patients for their basic care. Many recognize the need for additional training in primary care. Some integrated healthcare delivery systems are responding to that need. They are helping specialists obtain the retraining they need to handle primary-care business.

Old Paradigm	Between the Times	New Paradigm
Help physicians grow their practices, especially fee-for-service business	Help physicians track and hang on to managed-care business	Help physicians handle a panel of patients

Old Paradigm: Grow Physician Practices

Hospitals have developed numerous ways to help their physicians grow their practices. The logic is, the larger the physician practices, presumably the greater the amount of business for the hospital. The more the hospital does for physicians to help them grow their practices, presumably the more loyal the physicians will be to the hospital.

The following are some of the priority practices:

- Provide referrals for physicians through the physician-referral service.

- Provide opportunities and assistance to physicians in generating credible, free publicity through feature stories, press releases, and newsworthy events.

- Provide physicians with practice development services including practice audits, service excellence training, and patient satisfaction feedback systems.

- Work collaboratively with physicians to provide screening and health promotion services to the community, giving them exposure to key market segments and generating patient interest in them.

- Develop proactive speaker placement services, placing physicians before targeted groups in the community with presentations that feature them in a positive light.

- Stimulate professional referrals through nursing staff and other hospital staff members, using multiple tools of internal communication: sponsoring employee presentations, featuring physicians in employee newsletters, and featuring physicians in internal presentations concerning the quality of key clinical services.

- Nurses in particular have been known to make or break physician practices. They are a trusted, credible source of information about physicians for their friends and neighbors.

Between the Times: Attract Managed Care to Physicians

In a managed-care environment, physicians can gain or lose whole groups of patients if those patients change their insurance arrangements, and the physician doesn't participate in their new insurance arrangement. It makes sense, then, to aggressively inform the patient base of a physician about the physician's insurance plan participation so that employees don't lose the services of a physician simply because they overlook the connection between insurance plan and physician. Moreover, because patients choose their insurance arrangement anew every year, it is possible to get patients to come back to a practice—again, only if the physician informs those patients that they are welcome back and how to choose a plan that will allow them to come back.

Hospitals have been able, therefore, to help their medical staff members by developing form letters and software assistance so that physician practices can, in a timely way, keep their patient base informed about insurance arrangements and changes in insurance affiliations.

Moreover, hospitals help physicians be attractive to managed-care plans by providing them with ongoing information concerning their practice performance.

Finally, physicians look to a hospital and then to an integrated healthcare delivery system for assistance with contracting. Physicians don't want to be left out in the cold. In this period between the times, the market forces push physicians and hospitals to come closer together in the name of potential managed-care contracting.

New Paradigm: Patient Panels Management

In the new paradigm, the most important way to help physicians is to help them effectively handle a panel of patients. In a capitated arrangement, a physician is responsible for X number of covered lives. A family practice physician may, for example, be responsible for 2,500 covered lives. Those people relate to him as their personal physician. Obviously, if they all came to him on a given day or a given week or a given month, it would be impossible for him/her to meet their needs and handle the demand. In order to take care of the health needs of such a large group of people, the physician needs to reorganize radically the way he or she provides care. It makes sense, for example, for the physician to work much more collaboratively with a healthcare team of nursing and triage personnel so that requests from patients can be handled in the way that most appropriately meets their needs and uses resources.

The tools of informatics are pressed into service to assist the healthcare team in caring for a panel of patients. Reminders are sent to the panel of patients in a timely way concerning their annual check-ups or appropriate diagnostics, given their age and risk factors. The computer keeps a profile of the patients, and through appropriate software, develops such reminders in a timely way. Moreover, the profile of the individual patients' health promotion and screening needs is generated automatically at the time they come in for an appointment or a personal check-up.

A primary-care physician in a typical fee-for-service practice gets closest to patients that see him or her often. They become his "good patients." When handling a panel of patients, that attitude needs to change. The physician's satisfaction in caring for the sick shifts somewhat to a sense of satisfaction for not only caring for the sick, but aggressively helping patients stay well.

Henry Ford Health System, for example, has received grants from the Robert Wood Johnson Foundation that have been allowing them to construct various models for primary-care physicians working to handle a panel of patients.

Old Paradigm	Between the Times	New Paradigm
Satisfy primary-care physicians	Acquire primary-care physician practices	Free primary-care physicians from headaches that distract from patient care

Old Paradigm: Satisfy Primary-Care Physicians

In the more traditional world of fee-for-service marketing, an important priority for hospital leadership and hospital marketing is to work effectively with specialists to tune in to the needs of primary-care physicians and respond to them appropriately. If the specialist physicians don't adequately satisfy the primary-care physicians, the primary-care physicians will either look for a different place to practice, or in the case of a regional referral system, will refer patients to other regional tertiary-care providers.

The fundamentals of nurturing relationships with referring physicians are:

- *Identify a "hit list" of primary-care physicians* in a region whose business may be able to be shifted by more aggressive outreach and communication.

It is surprising to uncover the percentage of primary-care physicians in a region who change their referral patterns in a given year. A canard that turns out not to be true is that primary-care physicians are locked into their preferred specialists and consultants. It turns out that in a given market, 25 to 35 percent of specialty referral patterns are changed each year through a fairly standard set of causes:

- The primary-care physicians feel the specialists have taken their patients and not sent them back to them;

- The specialists have projected an attitude of superiority to the physicians or to the physicians' patients: "They've talked down to me;" and

- The specialist physicians didn't communicate adequately with the primary-care physicians; they didn't understand the primary-care physicians' need to be kept informed in a continuing way so that they could continue to support and respond to questions that their patients had of them.

In other words, the potential for generating additional referrals typically exists in a market if the specialists can be sprung from behind their walls and can begin to communicate effectively with referring physicians who are dissatisfied.

- *Develop within a specialty department agreed-upon protocols* for handling communications with primary-care physicians. Protocols should include:

  - The format and the timeliness of the written reports to primary-care physicians;

  - The timeliness of a phone call that adds a personal touch; and

  - The timeliness of the exam notes and medical records. These are all cues to primary-care physicians about whether or not their business is appreciated.

- *Provide specialists with ongoing qualitative insights from focus groups with primary-care physicians.*

  This allows them to fine-tune how they treat and respond to primary-care physicians. At times, the live feedback is so disturbing and embarrassing, that it prompts behavior changes by specialists who seemed irremediably stuck in their ways. They don't admit that they have been stung, but nonetheless, they change. Moreover, providing quantitative baseline and tracking information on primary-care physician satisfaction with their services helps them stay on top of their business.

- *Avoid the impression of a "resident run" service.*

  Make sure the attending physicians are actively, clearly involved in the patients' care and that care is not just turned over willy-nilly to residents.

- *Set up access systems* with specialty physicians that makes the challenge of getting a referral into a hospital easier.

  The famous phrase of the specialist, "I can always get a patient in for a doctor if the doctor calls me directly" betrays a kiss-of-death attitude. It says the referring doctors—if they go out of *their* way—can secure the services that they need. Instead, it becomes important to set up a whole system so that "one call handles it all."

- *Work to provide the right kind of continuing medical education (CME).*

Such programs can be designed and offered in a market-sensitive and market-driven way, or they can be set up in the traditional "expert/out" way. Asking the specialists what they want to present is not the first step of effective CME. Instead, ask the referring physicians what they want to hear and where and when they want to hear it.

For example, Indiana University Medical Center's Krannert Heart Institute developed a very successful market-driven CME program. With the help of a grant from a pharmaceutical company, they developed a "Family Practice Update" program for a specially invited group of primary-care physicians. Spaces for 50 physicians were reserved. In the course of a 2½-day institute, the faculty members presented the information about advances in heart disease that were of the most interest and the most use for family practice physicians. They mingled with the physicians during the breaks and during meals. Enough money was in the grant to have the physicians include their spouses in the trip to the Indianapolis area. The update was held at an attractive resort setting. A hands-on component was built into the update so that the physicians could learn for themselves some of the techniques presented, and could immediately apply them to their practices. This combination of hands-on learning and intensive training from a first-rate faculty, designed specifically for them, proved very attractive. All 50 slots were filled very quickly. Within the next week after the update, referrals came to the Krannert Institute from those physicians— referrals that they had never before received.

Continuing medical education, when designed in a market-based way, proves to be an important lever for generating additional referrals. Many primary-care physicians, when asked how they decide on a particular specialist, will say, "I heard him or her give a talk." By that they mean they had a chance to observe the physician up close and make judgments about their humanity and specialized skill. It's not any old talk that prompts such a response. It's a talk given well, authoritatively, and fresh for the primary-care physicians' ears.

Between the Times: Purchase Primary-Care Practices

Much of what has been learned concerning effective handling of primary-care physician relations continues to be valuable, of course, into the era between the times and even into the new paradigm. However, again because of market forces, hospitals and healthcare systems begin to place a heavy premium on making sure that primary-care physicians are indeed "locked in" as referral sources.

Increasingly, an attractive option for primary-care physicians who themselves are worried about their futures is to sell their practices, or at least the assets, to a hospital or a healthcare system. It is like an early retirement lump sum—without the retirement. Physicians typically are assured of making, in terms of a net margin, a similar amount of money as they made in private practice, but find that many of the worries and concerns of managing a practice are taken off their shoulders. When a hospital or healthcare system establishes an attitude of respect and collaboration, physicians do not feel that they have "sold out" their independence.

Many primary-care physicians, of course, maintain their independent identity, and at times, even their solo practices. But the selling option becomes more attractive than under the old paradigm. It gives some assurances to primary-care physicians that they will be part of a larger enterprise that will be able to survive in an era of managed-care contracting.

New Paradigm: Practice Management

Once primary-care physicians are practicing in a salaried environment, it is very important to actually relieve them of a lot of the cares that they had when they were running their own private-practice businesses. Hospitals and healthcare systems, therefore, need to develop expert practice management capabilities so that practices can be run more efficiently and effectively.

Physicians are free to concentrate on patient care through other initiatives from the healthcare system, such as the following:

- patient-care teams including nurses, physicians, and techs for handling panels of patients

- improved internal systems that shorten the times for patients moving through the healthcare continuum

- improved systems for arranging diagnostic tests and inpatient care

- Better turnaround time and communication from laboratory and X-ray departments

- Easier access to records

- More support in complying with managed-care and quality assurance dictates

All these steps can make life easier and more efficient for primary-care physicians working in the new paradigm.

Old Paradigm	Between the Times	New Paradigm
Information to physicians on their financial performance vis-à-vis the hospital	Information to physicians on their clinical performance vis-à-vis peers	Information to physicians on both their financial and clinical performance vis-à-vis benchmark performers

Old Paradigm: Information on Financial Performance

When hospitals shifted to the Medicare DRG system, it became very important for them to share information with physicians on physician practices concerning length of stay. Wide variations existed in most medical staffs between physicians, for one and the same diagnosis. Some physicians kept patients in the hospital much longer than others.

By sharing such information with physicians and demonstrating how much it was either benefitting or hurting the hospital, physicians, especially if they saw that information in comparison to the other members of their department, gradually began to change their practice patterns so that they wouldn't continue to be outliers. Such is the subtle power of peer pressure and objective information.

Between the Times: Information on Clinical Performance

As hospitals and physicians get ready for package pricing, they begin to study the pathways that patients take for a particular DRG and determine how to make the overall experience of care less costly while not diminishing the quality of the care. In order to make appropriate decisions, physicians need and depend upon accurate data not only about their financial performance but also on their clinical performance, so they can relate cost and quality, outcomes and resources utilized. Such information is best understood in comparison to similar information concerning their peers within the same department of the hospital.

New Paradigm: Information on Benchmark Performers

With physicians participating in capitated contract relationships, it becomes important to learn from other successful integrated healthcare delivery systems across the country. Some systems have been working within a capitated construct for much longer than others. Some have been more aggressive in managing both financial and clinical performance. Some have achieved rather remarkable results. It makes sense then to study examples of success and to compare one's performance to those benchmark performers.

MARKETING TO EMPLOYERS

Old Paradigm	Between the Times	New Paradigm
Networking	Carve out contracts	Full capitation

Old Paradigm: Networking with Employers

A natural affinity exists between hospital executives and other business executives in a region. They are practicing the same fundamentals of business, working within government rules and regulations, supplying jobs for the region, and depending on motivated employees for their success. Serving on hospital boards has been a badge of achievement and status for a business executive. For many years, it was a natural to have warm and cordial relationships with leading executives and business owners in the community. They were the source of some of the largest gifts to hospitals. Moreover, they served not only on the boards of directors but also to spearhead hospital capital campaigns.

As employers increasingly begin to be concerned about rising health-care costs and their rising healthcare benefit payments, the climate begins to change. Employers, while still positively disposed to hospitals as important resources for a community, begin to study ways to get a handle on rising healthcare costs. During this period, it makes sense for hospital leaders to aggressively nurture relationships with employers— to keep them informed about a hospital's efforts at cost containment, to keep them informed about advances at the hospital so that employers don't begin to turn on them as enemies or as sluggards in the fight to reduce healthcare costs.

It makes sense for a hospital, therefore, to host a continuing round of CEO roundtables, or high-profile breakfasts for business leaders. Such meetings provide a forum for employers and hospital leadership to share insights into what can be done or could be done in a given community. They begin to establish a climate for potential direct contracting between healthcare providers and employers. They also stimulate employers to talk with one another outside of the walls of the hospital.

Between the Times: Carve Out Contracts

When employers are ready to be more aggressive in terms of reducing their healthcare costs, they are open to overtures concerning fixed rates for some key clinical services. The higher ticket items to employers are the first ones to be offered or sought for direct, carve-out contracts such as open heart surgery, high-risk maternity, rehabilitation, and neurosurgery.

If a hospital has been successful in putting in place an active physician hospital organization, such contracts can be written to include hospital and physician fees—increasing satisfaction on the part of employers with the contract.

New Paradigm: Full Capitation

Employers are dissatisfied with the limits of discount medicine. They look for ways to control utilization, shift risk to providers, predict their healthcare costs in a given year, and shift incentives for providers to control costs. They are, at this point, ready for capitation arrangements and options.

Old Paradigm	Between the Times	New Paradigm
Build relations	Provide models of cost containment	Partner in benefit design

Old Paradigm: Build Relations

In the old paradigm, if a hospital is strongly preferred by people in the community, employers typically insist that those hospitals be part of the panels that insurance companies put together for contracting purposes. High-cost hospitals could, in effect, get away with being high cost as long as they maintained, through the community, pressure on employers to put pressure on insurance companies. In many markets, the hospitals that are perceived as the best hospitals are automatically included in the provider panels presented by insurance companies to employers to offer their employees. The insurance companies believe in offering their customers what they want.

Between the Times: Provide Models

As insurance companies begin to be more selective concerning their provider panels, they begin to weed out higher-cost providers. Enterprising providers at this point approach business coalitions with suggestions to work collaboratively on reducing healthcare costs.

The Midwest Business Group on Health, for example, sponsored a private program with a number of participating hospitals to bring down the average cost of open heart surgery at those hospitals across the metropolitan Chicago region. They succeeded in doing so. Participating hospitals looked good in the eyes of the employer community. The model stimulated other providers to follow suit.

New Paradigm: Partner in Benefit Design

Most employers still prize their healthcare benefits as a key management tool. They desire to keep their employees seeing healthcare benefits as benefits. They have no desire to be seen as punitive by their employees. Therefore, they typically want to maintain choice for their employees. They know that their employees equate choice with securing quality. As a result, point-of-service plans have become more and more popular. In the point-of-service plan, employees choose a package that stipulates that they can indeed go out of a network of providers, but will have to pay more out-of-pocket if they do so. That preserves at least a semblance of choice. Statistically across the country, employees that choose a point-of-service option, rarely go outside the network and rarely pay those increased out-of-pocket costs. In other words, the point-of-service option becomes a way station for employees moving into true managed care—while preserving the semblance of choice.

Once employers have chosen a few competitive integrated healthcare delivery system/insurance packages to present to their employees for their employees' final selection, those systems are wise to work collaboratively with the employers to design an offering that meets the preferences and needs of the employees. They will, for example, provide the employer with easily understood information concerning that set of providers' performance. Report cards become an important tool for helping the employer steer employees to the most cost-effective option. If they can give assurances to employees concerning the superior quality of the lower cost option, everybody wins.

MARKETING TO MANAGED-CARE COMPANIES: PPOS AND HMOS

Old Paradigm	Between the Times	New Paradigm
The more relationships, the merrier	Choose partners	Dance close

Old Paradigm: The More Relationships, the Merrier

For a number of years, most hospitals' managed-care relationship strategy has been rather simple. The more contracts and relationships, the better. It doesn't make sense to be excluded from any. It makes sense to be a preferred provider on everybody's panel. That way, one doesn't lose any business. Conversely, the managed-care companies are intent on having as many "quality" providers on their panels as possible—no reason for them to lose a relationship with an employer over a missing provider.

In such a setting, the managed-care companies can't really deliver on their promise to deliver volume to a provider because there are so many competitors in the market offering the same set of hospitals. It is hard for the managed-care companies to differentiate themselves. If they can't deliver on their promises of volume, it doesn't make sense for providers to give them too much by way of a discount incentive. This situation leads to a static competitive market.

Between the Times: Choose Partners

Gradually, both parties to the relationship begin to see the benefits of choosing more selectively. If the managed-care provider can select lower cost, yet still have a quality set of providers, and jettison the higher-cost providers without alienating any target employers, it can offer a more attractive price to employers and improve its competitive position. Vice versa, as certain managed-care companies gather momentum, providers begin to worry that they might be excluded from contracts with them and lose the loyalty of employees that choose a managed-care option that does not include them.

Hospitals and managed-care companies, therefore, begin to woo and waltz one another looking for the match that will bring them the most return in the marketplace. On the part of the managed-care companies, they begin to see that much more is at work than simply lower costs and prices on the part of providers. Some providers, they learn, are not very good partners. The only time they ever hear from them is at the time of negotiations to set rates for the year. Other providers, on the other hand, act as if they are in partnership with the managed-care companies. If, for example, patients have paperwork difficulties with a given provider, some providers understand that it is in their best interest to solve those paperwork dilemmas and make it easier and simpler for the patient, and therefore maintain the relationship between the patient and the managed-care provider/healthcare provider. Some hospital administrators are constantly on the phone with the managed-care providers looking for ways to strengthen the relationship in the eyes of their eventual customers, the employers, and the employees.

From the hospitals' perspective, they realize that some insurance companies give them a much better match in terms of a business partner. Some are much more strategic and rigorous in their implementation than others. Some do a much better job of resolving patient complaints than others.

Some project an exclusive interest in the bottom line. Others seem to be able to manage concerns for the bottom line with customer satisfaction. Some cultures match. Others are clearly in conflict.

Both parties to the relationship begin to understand that choosing one partner makes it less likely that they can work effectively with other counterparts. Gradually, the market will probably fractionate into clear-cut alliances between certain providers and insurance carriers and others. This typically is a protracted period of engagement as potential partners evaluate and weigh the risks and rewards of dancing close.

New Paradigm: Dance Close

The decision to work in a concentrated way with one or a few managed-care companies on the part of a set of providers means that they have judged their longer term good is through market concentration instead of through partial contributions from many sources. The first providers that select the strongest managed-care providers with whom to partner leave the others choosing more meager fare, and vice versa.

For awhile, more exclusive relationships do not necessarily sever relationships with other managed-care companies or providers. Even when providers launch their own competitive HMOs or PPOs, they still can maintain contracting relationships with others in the marketplace. Those relationships don't change until some see that it is in their best interest to jettison one company or another and concentrate on others.

Old Paradigm	Between the Times	New Paradigm
Stand-alone marketing	Stand-apart marketing	Co-marketing

Old Paradigm: Stand-Alone Marketing

In the old paradigm, hospital market and managed-care company market are two separate things. Each entity does its own marketing.

The hospitals marketed to secure patients. Managed-care companies marketed to secure additional enrollees.

Between the Times: Stand-Apart Marketing

Gradually, certain managed-care companies realize that they can have more of an impact on employees if they work with providers creatively to get in front of those employees. It's not typically enough to just compete with everyone else at the moment of enrollment. If a hospital with its clout can get inside a company and work with a managed-care company, for example, to put on a health screening or a series of educational, brown-bag presentations to employees earlier in the year, apart from the time of enrollment, the name of the managed-care option may be better known and at the top of employees' consciousness when they make their annual choice.

While the partners are still moving around one another, seeing if they want to work more consistently with one another on a more exclusive basis, there is time for multiple, cooperative, but separate marketing ventures. An insurance company may sponsor with a provider a major conference for women or a medical conference for referring physicians. The names of both established organizations appear as sponsors, but standing apart rather than as one.

New Paradigm: Co-Marketing

Once the die is cast and integrated healthcare delivery system has chosen an insurance partner or has developed its own competitive insurance product, the relationship then goes through further evolution. At first, the insurance provider is still determined to be able to contract with other providers, perhaps outside the immediate region. The network provided by a given system is rarely adequate for the objective of capturing X00,000 covered lives. Gradually, however, if both parties have chosen well and the provider system and the insurance provider have adequate clout in the marketplace, and are well perceived by the marketplace, there can be more synergy in clearly identifying with one another.

This is the time when budgets are combined, and the delivery system and insurance provider aggressively go after the market together.

Those who have predicted that the age of managed care will lead to less consumer marketing and less consumer advertising have not studied markets where HMOs are aggressively going after the market. The HMOs have larger ad budgets than hospitals have ever had.

In summary, it is important for healthcare marketers to understand where their markets stand in this time of transition—the amount of capitation, whether and how quickly employers will insist on capitation, how much fee-for-service business still exists, and how the purchase decisions are being made. With a clear understanding of these dynamics, healthcare marketers can decide what strategies and what combinations of old, new, and between the times strategies will produce the greatest results in the marketplace.

When everyone around them is confused and unsure about what to do to survive the future, healthcare marketing executives will be equipped to provide steady, surefooted leadership and counsel.

CHAPTER 2

Marketing an Integrated Healthcare Delivery System: The Fundamental Things Apply

INTRODUCTION

In this time of transition, healthcare executives are caught in an apparent contradiction.

Marketing an integrated healthcare delivery system is at first blush a daunting challenge. To make a household name out of something that currently has zero name recognition; is a very complicated product idea; is not only a new product but a whole new product category; and apparently has no immediate perceived benefit to the marketplace, appears to be an impossible challenge for a marketer.

On the other hand, it is ultra-important that the marketplace recognize and understand what an integrated healthcare delivery system is. Why? In the future, the market will be purchasing healthcare differently than it has in the past. In the past, people selected physicians and hospitals, and then had their healthcare paid for by their employers' insurance. In the future, people will be choosing a *whole package*— doctors, hospitals, other healthcare providers, and their insurance— in *one and the same choice*.

As difficult as the marketing challenge is, it can be done if we first recognize just how difficult a challenge it is; stop making it more difficult than it needs to be; and practice the fundamentals of effective marketing in a concentrated, committed way.

JUST HOW DAUNTING IS THE CHALLENGE?

I have a fear that healthcare leaders are going to soon turn to their marketing staffs and rather blithely commission them to market their newly minted integrated healthcare delivery systems. They will give the impression that they think the task is routine. They will give the impression that they think putting together an integrated healthcare delivery system was the *real* work. The marketing, in comparison, should be a piece of cake.

There is no doubt that putting together an effective integrated healthcare delivery system is a monumental organizational and political accomplishment. It means that the following has been accomplished:

- A group of hospitals has worked out past antipathies and succeeded in developing close working relationships so that they can, as a group, cover a geographic area and contract together.

- Physicians of all the medical staffs involved have come together and

  - are making cost-effective medical resource decisions;

  - understand how to work in a capitated environment; and

  - have resolved their control and fear issues and feelings.

- The full range of appropriate healthcare service settings—from home care, to intermediate care, to rehabilitation, to skilled nursing, to hospice—have been integrated and coordinated with a full range of inpatient and outpatient settings.

- A very active program of prevention, early detection, and health education has been launched.

- Appropriate insurance and underwriting capabilities or arrangements have been put in place, and all the back-office functions have been developed and are working smoothly.

There is no doubt that putting together a true integrated healthcare delivery system is a mammoth challenge and, when accomplished, a tour-de-force achievement. Anyone who pulls it off is a masterful leader and negotiator, a combination visionary and doer. That is why, as yet, there are so few true integrated healthcare delivery systems in existence. (An even more impossible commission will be for marketers who are asked to market integrated healthcare delivery systems that aren't yet real or able to demonstrate value and results. In this chapter, we are assuming that a true integrated healthcare delivery system has been established.)

As impressive a feat as it is from an organizational and management perspective, all that work and achievement is still only half the battle. Successfully marketing it, reaching the marketplace in such a way that the marketplace understands and is comfortable with an integrated healthcare delivery system, carries the same magnitude of difficulty as the establishment of the entity. After all the lawyers' opinions have been presented, multiple organizational charts drawn, and the endless task force meetings and planning retreats a memory, the work of bringing an integrated healthcare system to market begins.

Unless leadership first reflects on how hard the marketing challenge really is, it will never get accomplished.

I have a sense that the mood will be "we've done the hard part, now just tell the story." It will be similar to the cook of a Thanksgiving dinner who has organized, prepared, seasoned, and coordinated a big feast with many dishes and says to the invited guests "now just sit down and eat." We've done the hard part, all you marketers have to do is to invite people to come in and enjoy.

Why Is It Such a Difficult Marketing Challenge?

1) An integrated healthcare delivery system is a very complicated product idea. It puts together a number of things that the marketplace previously purchased separately. It is a solution to a number of things the market never knew were problems. For example, an integrated healthcare delivery system makes physicians, hospitals, and other healthcare providers into one organized entity. The marketplace, however, never realized that doctors were totally separate from hospitals. They always assumed that in some vague way doctors who are on staff at hospitals worked for the hospitals. They never understood the fact that the goals and the

financial incentives for the hospitals and physicians in the past were not one. In fact, they were often at odds.

Moreover, an integrated healthcare delivery system puts together the delivery of healthcare with insurance. Healthcare providers and insurance companies share the risk. The marketplace never understood or cared that providers and insurance companies weren't sharing the risk in the past.

2) Marketing an integrated healthcare delivery system is marketing not just a new product but a new product *category*. The marketplace has no previous handles for understanding it clearly. It calls, therefore, not just for a new product launch, but for a new product category launch. (The marketplace resisted something as straightforward and mundane as instant coffee until the resistances were understood. The introduction of an integrated healthcare delivery system is that much more difficult.)

3) There is currently zero recognition for the concept of an integrated healthcare delivery system. The marketing effort has to take people painstakingly up each rung of the ladder of marketing achievement, from awareness to understanding, to top-of-mind awareness, to preference, to trial. Any organization that has been through such a basic march up the marketing ladder knows that it is no small feat and that it requires great resources, commitment, and imagination. The marketing challenge is greater than the challenge of turning a low-profile, best-kept-secret hospital into one that is preferred and used by a given market. In a hospital marketing turnaround, at least the market knows what the product, a hospital, is. Marketing, therefore, can concentrate on differentiating a particular brand and doesn't have to first establish an understanding of the product.

4) There are no obvious ways to move from what is known to the unknown and to make the unknown, better known—the fundamental approach to marketing a service.

5) An integrated healthcare delivery system has been developed out of the product or production orientation and not out of a market orientation. The use of words like "seamless" and "gatekeeper" are a sure tip-off that healthcare leaders are talking to themselves and not taking into account the sensibilities of the marketplace.

6) The language itself is very tortured and not at all user friendly. An "integrated healthcare delivery system" is language that those on the inside, over time, can begin to understand. It is not a term that catches the ear or conveys luminous meaning to the marketplace.

7) The concept of an integrated healthcare delivery system is not yet articulated in terms of benefits to the marketplace. To this point, *features* are described and explained. How those features benefit the marketplace is not made clear.

In summary, when you have a new, very complicated product concept that the marketplace doesn't understand, expressed in language that is arcane, and you are starting with zero name recognition in a marketplace that is terribly cluttered—it is a very daunting marketing challenge indeed.

MARKETING INTEGRATED HEALTHCARE DELIVERY SYSTEMS WILL BE A NECESSARY TASK

Marketing the integrated health systems is, however, necessary—despite the problems and obstacles in the way—because integrated healthcare delivery systems are what customers will be purchasing in the future to take care of their healthcare needs. This represents a basic shift in the healthcare business paradigm.

Marketing at its heart is the management discipline that focuses on how purchase decisions are made. It is the art and science of choice. That is why marketing develops in the United States where there is free choice and then spreads to other parts of the globe where there are free-market economies. Tracing how decisions are made—what is chosen, by whom, using what decision variables, and at what weights—is the fundamental first step in effective marketing.

In the old paradigm,[1] people in need of healthcare chose physicians. Their physicians then chose the hospitals, and the patients' insurance paid for it all.

---

[1] The old paradigm still predominates in most areas of the country and will continue for quite some time until the managed-care proportion of the business reaches a tipping point of 35 to 40 percent. Then the markets move into the new paradigm relatively rapidly, as has been the case in Minneapolis.

In the new paradigm, Scenario #1, employers present two or more healthcare *packages* to employees to choose from. The competing packages include doctors, hospitals, other healthcare providers and settings, *and* the reimbursement or insurance arrangements all in one. If employees choose to receive care outside one of these packages, they pay substantial amounts of money out of their own pockets.

The new paradigm includes two scenarios. Scenario #1 describes a continuation of current market forces. In this scenario, employers make the selection among competing health system plans and present their selections to their employees. Employees then make the final selection.

This scenario of the new paradigm is one that is already occurring in markets with heavy managed-care penetration.

Scenario #2 will come to pass if any version of healthcare reform ever includes the idea of "regional purchasing cooperatives," which were featured in President Clinton's original version of reform. In this scenario, regional purchasing cooperatives make the selection among competing system plans and then present them to consumers for final selection. In this scenario, employers are out of the loop and consumers, a broader group than employees, make the final selection.

In most markets across the country, we are "between the times." The marketing rules and strategies for the most part still follow the old paradigm. We are still marketing physicians and hospitals to the largest part of the market, and marketing our "package" to a smaller portion of the market. Being "between the times" is a difficult situation to be in. It is difficult to gear up for two very different marketing and business challenges. The temptation is to fall into an either-or posture rather than a both-and one. This schizophrenia for hospital-based marketers is no different from the one physicians experience in their offices on a daily basis, as they handle pre-paid and fee-for-service patients at one and the same time. They say to the fee-for-service patient calling on the phone— yes, come in for a consultation. They have their nurse triage and counsel the pre-paid patients before telling them to come in to the office.

Most employers will still give their employees some choice. Most employers want to keep their employees happy. They typically start their selection process of managed-care plans with an understanding of where their employees prefer to go for their healthcare—if there are preferences in a given market. If costs are competitive, employers try to give employees a package that includes their preferred hospitals and doctors. Moreover, employers understand that for American workers, choice is tightly bound up with the issue of quality. In our culture, we believe if we have free choice, we will select quality. If there is no choice, if an employer gives only one healthcare insurance package option, there will, for employees, be a perceived decline in quality.

Therefore, comparatively few employers have felt it necessary to say to their employees, "Here is your one healthcare package—these doctors, hospitals, and coverage—take it or leave it. You have no choice."

Marketing an integrated healthcare delivery system is necessary because that is the new object of the health purchase decision. In either scenario of the new paradigm, the one that is currently beginning to play in the marketplace as a result of employer initiative or a scenario that may be introduced by healthcare reform, the result will be the same. The market will no longer purchase physicians and hospitals and other providers for their healthcare—which will then be paid for by their insurance plan. They will buy the whole package all at once.

When managed care in a capitated form comes heavily to a given market, one stops marketing hospitals and begins, of necessity, to market integrated healthcare systems.

Breaking Out of the Bind—Difficult but Necessary: Successful Marketing of an Integrated Healthcare Delivery System

If marketing an integrated healthcare delivery system is a daunting yet necessary task, how can we break out of this apparent bind? We can break out of the bind in two ways:

1) Don't make the marketing of an integrated healthcare delivery system more difficult than it needs to be.

2) Apply the powerful fundamentals of classic marketing to this new challenge.

Don't make the marketing of an integrated healthcare delivery system more difficult than it needs to be.

We don't need to market all the intermediate steps between a freestanding hospital and an integrated healthcare delivery system.

Most organizations will go through a series of organizational forms on their way to the real thing. It doesn't make sense to try and make each transitional organizational form a household name, when that transitional form will soon give way to another transitional entity. To make something a household word takes concentrated resources and consistent communication over time. The marketplace could end up scratching its collective head if it was receiving multiple, successive messages about multiple, successive organizational forms. Perhaps it's better to wait until the real thing is in place than to launch discrete marketing campaigns behind each transitional form.

For example, the first step towards becoming an integrated healthcare delivery system and away from freestanding hospital status, is the development of the "community healthcare system," a continuum of one-stop healthcare services: inpatient, outpatient, rehabilitation, step-down, skilled nursing, and home-care service components.

With such a continuum in place, the temptation of leadership is to trumpet the organization's accomplishment to the community. "Market us not as a hospital anymore, but as a 'community healthcare system.'" Should the CHCS be marketed? Is it wise to downplay the identity of the mainframe hospital? (That's pronounced "CHICKS" by those in the know.) Isn't that still the entity the market is purchasing and the door, in most cases, to the rest of the community healthcare system. When does the marketplace benefit from knowing about a community healthcare system? Why waste effort in marketing a community healthcare system if it will soon give way to another transitional entity anyway?

The next step towards an integrated healthcare delivery system is for a hospital to form some organizational alliance with physicians—in order to have adequate contracting capabilities and to tackle health resource decisions and cut costs. Is the resulting PHO what should be marketed to employers and the community? After all the effort that goes into creating a successful PHO, it is understandable that participants want the community to recognize the achievement—but again, is it what should be marketed to employers and the community? In many situations, PHO members soon realize that this organizational structure is also a transition to one that will more adequately match the needs of the marketplace. In larger markets, one hospital or community healthcare system and PHO isn't enough to satisfy the needs of employees and employers. Typically, a large employer has employees across a large geographic area, and one local hospital and its localized physician group isn't an adequate contracting partner.

For example, one midwestern hospital/community healthcare system/PHO was all set to launch a major marketing effort behind its PHO. The hospital had spent millions purchasing assets of physician practices, enlisting active members, structuring a 50/50 control relationship with the physicians, and contracting with a range of specialists.

They stopped the marketing effort, however, when employers told them that they wouldn't contract with them as they were then organized. The employers' employees thought too highly of a competitive tertiary care hospital in the same market. Unless they came to negotiations *with* that other hospital/PHO, they were dead in the water. They went out and formed an alliance with the tertiary-care hospital and its PHO— formerly a competitor and now a partner.

The third intermediate entity, therefore, is the broader healthcare alliance/multi-hospital system/PHO organization. Is *this* then what should be marketed—or is it too a transitional organization?

In the St. Louis area, for example, is the Barnes/Jewish/Christian system what should be named, branded, and aggressively marketed? Or should the new entity delay its marketing campaign until it has a strong *insurance* capability in place, and then name, brand, and market the whole package?

We don't have to make our marketing challenge harder than it needs to be by putting too much effort into marketing each transitional form on the way to the real thing. The decision of which organizational form to concentrate on depends on how quickly change will come in a given market, the strength of one's name in the market, competitors' momentum, and the likelihood of the delivery system remaining separate from insurance.

Avoid Using Industry Jargon in Our Marketing.

We don't need to make our job harder by automatically using healthcare industry language in our communications. At times, healthcare lingo is confusing. At times, misleading. At times, offensive.

We make our job harder when we use insider language instead of straightforward, easy-to-understand consumer language. Take, for example, the term "gatekeeper" to describe the role of the primary-care physician. It's industry language to express, in a shorthand way, the primary-care physician's role in retarding the flow of unnecessary referrals to specialists. It's not, however, the way we want to communicate the important role of the primary-care physician in the new era. "Gatekeeper" conjures up images of sheep being led, perhaps to slaughter. The gatekeeper says yay or nay. Some will be allowed in. Others will be held back. Such a term depicts the primary-care physician in a punitive and negative way. We can instead use consumer-friendly terms such as "guide," or "advocate through the system." A guide does at times play the role of steering a charge away from harm—unnecessary utilization is ultimately bad for the client, not just the system—but a guide's first purpose is a safe and satisfying journey.

Another insider term is the word "system"—as used in "Community Healthcare System" and "Multi-Hospital System."

The term "system" is so overused in popular culture as to be practically empty of meaning. Everything is described as a system—drinking water system, total work-out system, pet food system, water bed system—until the term almost has no meaning.

A term made popular by the fields of cybernetics and computers, it refers to an interactive set of relationships with feedback and self-corrective loops. As used to describe healthcare organizations, however, it strikes consumers as impersonal, cold, and mechanistic.

That's why many healthcare organizations are beginning to change their names to more open-ended and personal ones. For example, Evangelical Health Care System has renamed itself after merging with the Lutheran General System, Advocate Health Care. St. Mary's Hospital evolved into—not St. Mary's Health Care System—but St. Mary's Health Services.

A final example of a term that has become very popular within the industry but which can, if used willy-nilly, make the communications challenge more difficult than it needs to be, is the term "seamless," as in "seamless healthcare delivery system." "Seamless" can say to an outsider—no fingerholds, monolithic, "how do you find your way into it?" The term is supposed to express something quite different, of course—namely, the patient will move in a timely way from the more-expensive to the less-expensive setting without a perceived break in service.

Using healthcare insider language can distance us from the consumer and put us in a hectoring, lecturing, "educating" mode instead of in the classic mode of sound marketing—namely, understanding the market's perceptions and needs and designing the product to respond to those needs.

Apply the powerful, fundamental approaches of authentic marketing to this new challenge

1) Trace how the purchase decision is made.

2) Reposition the concept of an integrated healthcare delivery system in terms of consumer benefits.

3) Rework the product and place "P"s of the marketing mix to mirror the consumer benefits.

4) Take charge of the system's identity.

5) Orchestrate a communications campaign.

Trace How the Purchase Decision Is Made.

The first powerful, fundamental tactic of classic marketing is to understand as completely as possible how the purchase decision is made. That understanding will reveal many insights into how to influence that purchase decision.

To understand the purchase decision includes understanding the following:

- who is choosing, and their profiles;
- if more than one decisionmaker, the sequence of decisions and the degree of influence the decisionmakers have on one another;
- the decision variables used in the decision; and

- the relative weight of the decision variables.

The variables they will use, given what we currently know about how consumers choose health plans, will mostly likely be:

- the plan their physicians belong to;

- the size of the premium they will have to pay out of pocket;

  Some people will stay with their physician even though they have to pay a substantial out-of-pocket premium. Others are ready to switch as soon as the out-of-pocket premium appears too great. Price sensitivity analyses will reveal where the price breaks are in a given population and at what point price becomes more important than maintaining physician ties.

- convenience—geographically and in terms of access; and

- reputation for quality—in terms of both clinical expertise and service.

  Each of these variables play against one another depending on their intensity—e.g., very high reputation for quality makes the need to travel a few extra miles less distasteful, whereas across the street convenience with a good, not necessarily great, reputation for quality will be acceptable.

The following are implications of the new paradigm decision model:

- Physicians are now part of the package that the consumer is choosing. Physicians are no longer the intermediate decisionmaker for the consumer.

- The larger the primary-care physician panel, and the better the participating physicians—both in terms of practice patterns and loyalty from their patients—the stronger the edge one system will have over another.

- Reputation for quality, both in terms of clinical excellence and service, continues to be important in the new paradigm—as it was in the old. Traditional high-tech product line appeals, however, have to be used carefully because they can backfire if they end up with "adverse selection," i.e., a higher proportion of sick or high-risk members in the system plan.

- The more complete the geographic coverage, the fewer losses in the selection process from those who make the decision based on convenience.

- If there is perceived parity between competing systems, the selection will be based on other, next-in-line variables than the ones listed above. If price, quality, and convenience are perceived as equivalent, next-level variables will determine the decision for key segments.

  - One segment will ask, for example, "Which system will best satisfy women with specific healthcare needs?"

  - Men who know they are at risk for heart disease will ask, "Which is the best hospital if I ever have heart problems?"

  - Another segment, expecting a baby, will ask "Which is the best hospital at which to have a baby?"

  The marketing program in this situation needs to target distinct demographic and need segments within the general consumer population.

- *Consumers* make the final choice and are the real focus of marketing—after the organizing and negotiating hurdle has been jumped. Systems will have to compete for the attention and loyalty of the general populace. The mind of the consumer is the place where the battle will be won or lost. The system that best differentiates itself and penetrates consumer consciousness is the one that ultimately wins.

- Women are the key target for marketing. Women will continue to be the decisionmakers for themselves and their families. They will continue to take the lead role in the selection of plans. Understanding how they are choosing between competing systems and plans will be very important in the design of effective marketing strategies.

Reposition the Concept of an Integrated Healthcare Delivery System in Terms of Consumer Benefits.

Notice how all the terms in the phrase "integrated healthcare delivery system" are expressed from the *provider's* point of view. The second marketing task is to recast the product in terms of consumer benefit to determine what needs reworking about the product and place "P"s of the marketing mix, as well as to make the promotion more effective.

integrated—A term expressed from the standpoint of the provider who has integrated the system.

healthcare delivery—Again, seen from the standpoint of the provider who does the delivery.

system—All the parts of the provider's offering relate to one another.

The following are the fundamental benefits to the consumer of an integrated healthcare delivery system:

Consumer benefit #1: Lower costs with the same, or improved, quality of care

All the components of an integrated healthcare delivery system point to the same need. They all contribute to lowering the costs of healthcare by taking out the unnecessary costs that result from system design.

Taking out the unnecessary costs that are due to the design of the system means the system can cost less *without a dilution or lowering of the quality of care*. These costs are not part and parcel of delivering quality care. Those with a total quality management background can understand that lower costs can produce, if achieved through system design changes, higher quality.

Five changes in the system work together to produce this apparently abracadabra benefit:

1) Fee-for-service gives way to capitation. Providers don't get paid for each thing they do, they are paid to orchestrate the care of a given population. That change in turn leads to an urgent redirecting of energies and realignment of motivations.

   If hospitals and doctors in a capitated system don't bring costs down, there won't be anything left over at the end of the year from their capitation grant, which is a fixed amount of income. No marching together, no margin for anyone.

   The truism of the previous paradigm, "No margin, no mission," is turned on its head. "No mission, no margin."

2) Keeping people healthy is a direct way to save resources. Keeping them healthy keeps them out of expensive inpatient stays.

3) Physicians reexamine their health resource decisions—especially those made in the most expensive setting of all, the hospital. Hospital administrators can't save the system much—once they are lean and mean and downsized. Huge savings, however, can come from physicians reexamining how they routinely make their health resource decisions. Hence, the development of critical paths.

4) Healthcare settings are developed to match, as inexpensively as possible, the needs of the recovering patient. Acute care is supplemented with the full array of outpatient, rehab, and home-care services. Move patients to the less costly setting as soon as appropriate—lower costs without loss of quality.

5) Case management makes sure there is a care plan for each patient, monitors the patient's progress through the healthcare system, convenes appropriate resources in a timely way, and makes sure there are as few unnecessary steps, and therefore costs, in the patient's experience as possible. In these ways, case management produces lower costs and improved quality.

Consumer benefit #2: An easier experience for the patient

An integrated healthcare delivery system promises a much easier, less anxiety-producing experience for a patient needing care.

No matter which part of the system patients first enter, the one who greets them is knowledgeable about the whole system and can guide and direct them in a way that renders simple what otherwise would be quite complex. Paperwork is simplified. A patient registers once instead of each time she/he enters a new part of the system. Data about the patient are accessible throughout the system.

Patients' medical records follow them. There is no need, therefore, for multiple workups and case histories or duplication of tests.

Consumer benefit #3: A simplified judgment of quality

Potential patients don't have to conduct extensive, separate research studies to determine if each and every physician and care setting they may encounter in the course of an illness is first rate or not.

If they know and trust the sponsoring organization, they can trust that the organization has done the checking and credentialing for them.

The one brand name gives them assurance of quality for all the parts. Patients can concentrate on getting well and don't waste energy on multiple evaluative purchase decisions.

One purchase decision does it all.

Looking at an integrated healthcare delivery system through the eyes of the customer forces attention on the aspects of the integrated healthcare delivery system that may otherwise receive short shrift. That leads to the third fundamental of classic marketing.

Rework the Product and Place "P"s of the Marketing Mix to Mirror the Consumer Benefits.

In order to demonstrate lower costs with improved quality, the system needs to be able to provide meaningful information, in a before-and-after format—especially to employers so they can communicate the facts to their employees—concerning reductions in costs and improvements in quality that result from collaborative system design changes.

Such information is not an afterthought. The information system that produces such data is not something to be developed after the integrated healthcare delivery system is put in place. Such information systems are a constituent part of what an integrated healthcare delivery system is. Without this information there is, in effect, no integrated delivery system that is meaningful to the market. An integrated healthcare delivery system doesn't really exist until this information exists. Don't bother marketing it, therefore, if the consumer benefit that makes the whole thing meaningful can't be met.

The integrated healthcare delivery system will not deliver on its promise to the market unless it can deliver on the promise of an easier experience. Henry Ford Health System in Detroit, for example, has been concentrating for the last five years on the internal issues that have to be resolved for a system to function as a system. These issues include: one-time registration into the system; knowledgeable, first-encounter staff members; portable patient records; and effective case management. Ford recognizes that the organizational structures are not what makes a system meaningful to the market. The system's ability to provide the benefits sought by the customer is what makes the system marketable. These elements are every bit as important a part of the product itself as the PHO, the nursing homes, the multi-hospital settings, and the HMO under the Ford organizational umbrella.

Take Charge of the System's Identity.

A clear, trusted, vibrant brand name responds to the "simplified judgment of quality" consumer benefit.

In the new era, multi-hospital/institutional systems need—in a way they didn't in the old paradigm—a centralized marketing function that jealously guards, advocates, and builds the system brand.

In the old paradigm, marketplace dynamics dictated keeping the corporate or central marketing function weak and making the marketing functions at the local hospitals and institutions strong. The purchase decisions concerning an individual hospital, or nursing home, or chemical dependency program, etc., were made by the doctors, discharge planners, and consumers at the local level. It made sense then for marketers to be decentralized, aggressively working at the purchase decisions where they were being made. In the new era, with a larger and larger share of the business locked in through contracts with a system, the balance has shifted. The system or corporate marketing function comes first.

*Taking charge of the system's identity begins with the development of a clear **positioning statement** and strategy.*

Unlike a mission statement, which articulates what an organization wants to be, the positioning statement articulates how the organization wants to be *perceived*. Mission statements run paragraphs, even pages, long. A positioning statement is one or two sentences long. It is the "take" on the organization that leadership wants the market to have.

An effective positioning statement arises out of three force fields— how the organization is currently perceived vis-à-vis competitors, what the real strengths and animating values of the organization are, and what the marketplace is looking for. Consequently, the hallmarks of an effective positioning statement are as follows:

- It differentiates the organization from competitors;
- It taps what is real about the organization and valued by the staff; and
- It responds to a felt need in the marketplace.

The first step, therefore, in taking charge of a system's identity is for leadership to hammer out and agree upon a positioning statement. That one- or two-line statement of self-identity is never used in communications to the outside. It serves rather as a platform for and check on all subsequent communications. The way the positioning statement is expressed to the outside world is through a consistently utilized name and themeline and a well-orchestrated identity campaign.

For example, the positioning statement for a major Midwest healthcare system reads:

> *We want to be perceived as the Healthcare System in our area that is so organized around patients' needs that, no matter what the point-of-entry into the System, patients feel secure and enfolded in care. Moreover, the System will be recognized as providing the finest array of physicians in the area.*

A positioning statement provides the whole organization—all the staff, employees, volunteers, and supporters who have such powerful word-of-mouth communication power—with a clear sense of direction and self-identity. Without it, an organization can waffle in multiple directions at once. Without it, the organization will continue to be bland and amorphous to the outside, instead of presenting a sharp, clear identity profile. Moreover, without a guiding positioning strategy, all those within the organization will continue to ask the legitimate "just who are we," self-identity question.

The exercise of developing a positioning statement, "What do we want the market to say about us in twelve months?" forces leadership to make some choices. The positioning statement highlights the attributes of the organization that will receive priority attention and resources and that will be most prominently featured in all communications.

After developing a positioning statement, the next step in taking charge of the system's identity is to select or confirm a name for the system.

More and more often systems must reassess their names for marketability. Especially after expanding to incorporate additional members or after merging with another system, it's time to revisit, for the sake of brand identity, the name of the system.

The options for approaching the renaming of a system are:

• Roll over the name of the lead historical Sponsor.

In many situations, the system in large part has actually been in existence for a number of years, but has been a background not foreground presence. This is particularly true for systems sponsored by religious organizations. The decision is often made to keep the name of the historical sponsor but to bring it into the foreground. Some examples are Adventist Health System, Franciscan Health Care, Baptist Health System, or Carondolet Health System.

- Select a geographic-oriented name.

For example, Intermountain HealthCare, Health Midwest, or Allegheny Health Care.

- Use the name of the most prominent member organization as the name of the system.

For example, Rush-Presbyterian, Baylor Health Care System, or The Johns Hopkins Health System.

- Select a name that conveys some benefit to the marketplace either in a direct or indirect way.

For example, Multicare, HealthOne, Servantcor, or UniHealth.

- Use phonemes to construct an appropriate name.

Given the number of names already taken and copyrighted by existing health organizations, many turn to manufactured names, ala Acura. For example, Inova or Sentara.

It is important—in order to avoid the kind of fiasco United Airlines found itself in after changing its name to Allegis—to test key sectors of the market's reactions to alternative names.

Conduct market research to assess whether the name conveys the meaning intended, to determine if the market hears anything negative in the name, and whether it's a believable and positive name.

Take charge of the names and signage of the organizations within the system.

Many multi-hospital systems across the country have oscillated over the last few years on the need to feature the name of the system more prominently than the names of their member organizations.

In the new era, names of system members will need to be changed. Each institution under the corporate umbrella that has a name totally unrelated to the name of the system, will need to be changed as marketplace dynamics dictate. For example, Cottage and Wyandotte Hospitals in the Ford System will be renamed Ford Cottage and Ford Wyandotte. Signage will need to be changed. The common decision to insert the name of the system on signage in a subordinate way, will need to be revisited.

The relationship of the member organization and sponsoring system is reversed in all signage and graphic standards. Instead of the member organizations appearing in the prominent, bold-faced position, and the system appearing in a subordinate lowercase position, the name of the system brand comes first and the name of the local manifestation of the brand comes second.

ST. MARY'S HOSPITAL

A Member of Mercy Healthcare

MERCY HEALTHCARE

St. Mary's Hospital

The most powerful tools for increasing or changing name recognition are buildings—visible from automobiles on traffic arteries—with big clear signs on them proclaiming their identity to motorists passing by. Prominent, well-identified buildings on traffic arteries are more powerful and efficient tools of communication than thousands spent on print or broadcast media. A system desiring increased brand identity makes all its buildings speak one franchise-enhancing message. Henry Ford Health System, for example, at this point is clearly perceived by the public as "more than a hospital." The main contributor to this achievement is the network of 30 large physician office buildings scattered throughout the Detroit market with the name Ford in big lighted letters.

After the positioning statement and name decisions comes the development of the themeline. The themeline works with the name to convey the chosen positioning to the market.

The name denotes the system and conveys what it is. The themeline connotes and adds an emotional charge to the name, expressing the narrative positioning statement in a packed, emotion laden way.

A good themeline should strike resonant chords in the organization while stretching the organization beyond its current performance.

Taking charge of the system identity means finally, using existing elements within the system for their full halo effect.

For example, a well-regarded hospital within the system can have very important halo effects for the system. At times, the reputation of the hospital is so strong that it will pull employees making their annual health plan decision to choose the system or plan of which the hospital is a part. In such a case, it is hard not to use synecdoche in the naming decision—i.e., naming the whole after a part. It is difficult to imagine the Jewish, Christian, Barnes merger not keeping in its new name some of the magic of the Barnes name.

Other component parts of a system with the power to influence employee decisions, which can be mixed and matched by leadership taking charge of identity dynamics, are:

- A fine obstetrics service. Young adults, a prime target for a system because of their more positive health status, oftentimes choose their plan based on where it will put them for delivering a baby.

  Young couples are known to switch out of one plan in order to deliver at the hospital of their choice and to switch back again to the original plan after the baby comes.

- A well-recognized heart program has pulling power, at least as a tie-breaker for employees reviewing competing systems and plans.

- A panel of excellent, well-regarded primary-care physicians can very directly influence employee choice of a system plan. For many, it is the most important, first-cut issue, i.e., whether their doctor participates in the system or not.

Taking charge of the system identity requires selecting and featuring the elements within the system that have built-in positioning power.

Orchestrate a Communications Campaign.

Taking a campaign approach to communicating the message of an integrated healthcare delivery system begins with four assumptions about the nature of communications in a crowded marketplace and incorporates two features peculiar to healthcare communications to achieve success.

The four assumptions are:

1) A campaign requires an umbrella strategy broad enough to allow a richness of subordinate themes and stories but clear enough to make the multiple messages—facets of one overriding theme—the strategic positioning.

2) Taking a campaign approach calls for well-calculated repetition of a message, in sufficient measure, to break through the clutter in the marketplace.

3) Taking a campaign approach allows advertising and public relations to be planned together and to work together to multiply the impact of each.

4) Taking a campaign approach means selecting themes and stories for their specific weight and gravity—selecting those that carry and convey the positioning and not selecting others just because they are newsworthy.

Two distinctive features of healthcare communications are:

1) Healthcare decisions are heavily influenced by word-of-mouth communication networks.

2) Women are the primary target of healthcare communications because women make the great majority of healthcare provider and insurance choice decisions.

The four assumptions about the nature of communications in a crowded marketplace:

1) Taking a campaign approach calls for an umbrella communications strategy broad enough to allow a richness of subordinate themes and stories, but clear enough to make all the multiple messages, facets of one overriding theme, the strategic positioning.

Take, for example, the campaign of Kaiser Permanente launched in 1987 and continuing as a platform campaign even today. The campaign theme "Good People, Good Medicine" is conveyed in a television series of commercials depicting attractive, caring, approachable primary-care physicians. Every year, another three or four physicians are selected from across the Kaiser System for these profiles to keep the campaign fresh. These television spots, done out of the corporate office, are available to and utilized by each of the Kaiser regions and supplemented and reinforced by regional print and public relations initiatives.

The platform campaign developed out of the market research Kaiser did—almost a decade ago—that indicated the public's major concern with HMOs in general, and Kaiser in particular, is that a member doesn't have a personal, ongoing relationship with a family doctor and as a result becomes lost in a huge, impersonal bureaucracy. The campaign is designed to answer that concern and nail the strategic positioning for Kaiser.

Kaiser wants to be known as "a stable, resource-filled organization that offers comprehensive care and coverage and a personal relationship with a family physician."

Taking a campaign approach allows an umbrella strategy that builds in flexibility for local issues and approaches while drawing all the subordinate stories back to the central communication challenge for Kaiser—namely, reinforcing what the market knows and finds attractive about Kaiser (that it offers comprehensive coverage and an impressive range of services and facilities) while hammering away at the market's central misgiving: loss of a personal relationship with a physician. "Good People, Good Medicine" says: "yes, Kaiser stands for good, stable medicine, but it also stands for friendly, approachable caregivers." Kaiser has not only selected the franchise it wants in the mind of the marketplace, Kaiser also knows that building that franchise takes a long-term commitment and consistent, coherent communications, i.e., a campaign.

2) Taking a campaign approach calls for well-calculated repetition, in sufficient measure, to break through the clutter in the market.

Having a penetrating positioning strategy is not enough to get the message about an integrated healthcare delivery system across. Neither is clever, compelling advertising enough to get the message across. Brilliant insight, and compelling flash and fire have to be coupled with the slow trod of sheer repetition of the message to be successful. People in our culture of mass communications have developed impressive abilities not to notice. If we let every communications message that washes over us every day register in our minds, our minds would short circuit. We only let through either what we are actively looking for (we notice refrigerator ads every 10 years, when we are looking for a refrigerator) or what breaks through our defenses.

Excellent creative has to be coupled with adequate exposure, reach, and frequency to have any effect. Energy and mass are required together for impact. It is estimated that it takes between six and eight coordinated exposures to a given market to even be noticed by that audience.

Just when the sponsor of a message is getting bored by a particular ad is just the time the market is, no doubt, first noticing it.

Out of this basic fact about the nature of communications in a crowded marketplace arises the role of the media planning professional, the person who calculates which set of communication vehicles will most efficiently reach—with adequate reach and frequency (CPM, or Reach per Thousand Population)—a given target audience.

The advertising community, of course, recognizes the importance of well-planned repetition, but it is not clear that healthcare leadership is always conscious of its importance. It is better to invest nothing on communications than to not execute a well-orchestrated campaign. Any one-shot mailing or set of sporadic print ads are hardly likely to break through the market clutter. Such efforts are, in effect, throwing resources down the drain. If a message is important to communicate to the market, as the message about an integrated healthcare delivery system surely is, then it is better to save and garner sufficient resources to invest in doing it right and well.

In a mid-size market, using television, print, and radio in a coordinated campaign to achieve adequate reach and frequency— say a gross rating point figure of 125 to 150 over two 8-week media flights—requires an investment running in the hundreds of thousands of dollars. In a major urban market, such a campaign will cost in the seven figures.

If an organization is not ready to make such an investment to achieve adequate reach and frequency with its media, it probably makes more sense not to spend anything at all.

3) Taking a campaign approach to communicating the message concerning an integrated healthcare delivery system means that advertising and public relations can be planned and executed in a way that magnifies, even multiplies, the impact of each.

One system, for example, planned to use a credible celebrity spokesperson in its advertising campaign, thinking that one effective way to communicate a rather complicated, new message is to have a trusted public figure take the public through it. The spokesperson not only appeared in the paid advertising, he was taken on a well-planned and executed spokesperson publicity tour as well. He was interviewed by almost all of the local news and talk shows. Clips of the paid advertising spots were used by the news programs as part of their news stories. As a result, total air time for the message secured through the public relations campaign equalled the air time purchased for the advertising. Planning the public relations and advertising together as two parts of the same campaign—with an eye towards one method feeding off the other, instead of each going off in different directions— doubled the impact of each. When public relations is put in tandem with advertising, in one coordinated campaign, the public relations becomes a little less spontaneous and opportunistic, but much more strategic. The stories to be placed are evaluated not just for the amount of air time or print space secured but also for whether or not they express the chosen positioning strategy. Quality *and* volume.

Conversely, by insisting that the advertising be done with an eye for what the media find newsworthy, advertising is pushed to be so on target with the needs of the market that even the non-paid media will want to pick it up and repeat it.

4) Finally, taking a campaign approach works with the assumption that, of the many themes and stories emerging from across an integrated healthcare delivery system, some will more adequately convey a chosen positioning strategy than others. Linking the positioning with the best themes and stories is at the heart of a successful campaign. Getting the whole organization inside the challenge of identifying the themes and stories that have the two-sided merit of not only expressing the positioning but also immediately appealing to the marketplace, pays off in many ways.

It does little good if a story expresses the positioning but does so in a didactic, or esoteric way. "Get the press to do a story on our vertically integrated healthcare system." Conversely, it will not serve the purposes of the communications campaign if a given story has natural appeal to the market but doesn't express the positioning strategy.

Take, for example, the system that made the story of its clinic for pregnant, unmarried teenagers one of the touchstones of its positioning as "a current embodiment of the next generation of healthcare." "More cost-effective healthcare, not through lowering quality standards, but through intelligent leveraging of resources."

The hospital and its entire obstetric staff, on a rotating basis, provided the clinic to the community on a sliding payment scale. It had such a positive reputation in the minority community that pregnant, unmarried teens were linked very early with excellent prenatal care. As a result, not only had the infant mortality rates plummeted in that community, but the number of low birth weight, million dollar babies resulting from inadequate prenatal care had plummeted as well.

The hospital, through the community clinic, demonstrated how the costs of healthcare to society could be lowered dramatically through an investment of resources where they can do the most good. In this case, costs of healthcare were lowered, and at the same time, health outcomes improved, through a system of providers—hospital, physicians outreach workers, clinic, and home health agency—using their skills and resources in a coordinated way.

Saving babies' lives is an inherently interesting story. That's what gives the story an immediacy of appeal. What makes it expressive of the positioning strategy is that babies were saved while reducing society's healthcare bill. To decrease the number of million dollar babies is to decrease the infant mortality rate. Healthcare costs are reduced while improving quality and doing good—which is precisely how the system wanted to be thought of by the marketplace.

Such a story in the previous paradigm of healthcare decisionmaking would not typically have been selected for a communications campaign. In the old paradigm, the freestanding hospital would position itself as a quality hospital through stories of its high-tech prowess; its specialized services such as open heart surgery or comprehensive cancer centers; and through its high-profile, trained-at-the-best-schools specialists. In fact, a story about a free OB clinic might have been rejected precisely because it conveyed the wrong message and might attract more of the "wrong" kind of customers.

With a shift in the healthcare decisionmaking paradigms comes the need for very different positioning strategies and a whole new crop of themes and stories with specific weights and gravities for carrying those positioning strategies.

Another system, for example, made the story of family practice a centerpiece expression of its positioning strategy.

Most people have little specific understanding of what a family practice physician is, what their training is about, or how they differ from other specialties. Through its research, the system recognized what kind of physician the market was looking for: one who takes a lasting, personal interest in the patient, one who understands the effects of disease on body, mind, spirit, as well as society; one who would quiet the patient through the healthcare maze in the event of a serious illness; one who answers questions and engages the patient as an adult; and one who is there through life's stages and ages. These qualities are precisely what the family practice specialty is designed to be. By telling the story of family practice, the system would in effect make it easier for the market to search out its excellent, extensive panel of family practice physi-cians—a larger, better-trained panel than competitive systems. Furthermore, the campaign aimed to make their family practice physicians a top-of-mind issue when employees were making their selection of a provider/insurance package.

If the market remembers the story, "family practice," and associ-ates all those positive attributes with this particular system, the system will have a distinct identity, separating it from the herd, and the market will have one, clear valuable reason for selecting this system/package over others.

A successful communications campaign not only works out of the above four assumptions about the nature of communications in a crowded marketplace, it also incorporates the distinctive attributes of communications in healthcare.

The two attributes distinctive to healthcare communications:

1) Healthcare decisions depend heavily on word-of-mouth communications.

   In a much more fundamental way than consumer product purchase decisions, healthcare decisions are heavily dependent on word-of-mouth communication networks. Below are some examples:

   • Busy primary-care physicians recognize that 80 to 90 percent of their patients come to them from the recommendations of other patients.

   • Newcomers to a neighborhood ask their neighbors for recommendations concerning doctors and hospitals, and the market-shares of the hospitals end up matching these neighborhood testimonial patterns.

   • Choices of alternative insurance options for employees are heavily influenced by conversations among employees about their experiences and preferences.

   • Consumers ask other healthcare professionals, especially nurses, for recommendations and appraisals of specialists. Nurses can make or break specialists' practices—at least in the old paradigm.

   The most productive results will be achieved by a campaign that taps into, influences, and even mobilizes these word-of-mouth networks. One large, important network that a healthcare system can tap into, influence, and mobilize—if it makes the effort—is its own "family" of employees, volunteers, vendors, and supporters. They have a more active stake in the outcome of the campaign and can be reached less expensively and more efficiently than other word-of-mouth networks. They number in the hundreds and thousands, and they are seeded throughout the market.

   Any positioning campaign starts here. Before going public, a system should take great pains to make sure every employer, physician, volunteer, board member, donor, and vendor understands and is ready to repeat and expand upon the system's positioning strategy.

One system, for example, launched a comprehensive campaign to its own "family" before launching its campaign to the general public. Leadership wanted the 10,000 employees, volunteers, and physicians to be ready—once the media campaign began—to answer questions from their friends and neighbors, and further, to be equipped to say "let me tell you more."

The internally focused campaign consisted of a direct-mail flyer from the CEO of the system to each employee and volunteer's home. It previewed and explained the upcoming public campaign; a pre-launch employee party; continuous-loop runnings of the campaign broadcast for all staff and shifts; an employee and volunteer contest tie-in with the campaign; and free giveaway promotional items, from cups to banners to fanny packs, featuring the new theme line and identity. A portable slide show presentation on the positioning strategy and campaign was developed for use in individual departmental meetings.

As a result of the internal campaign, employees and volunteers not only were not surprised when the external campaign hit and did not feel like outsiders looking in, they felt included and much more positively ready to face the coming era of change and reform.

The short course in the positioning strategy revealed to employees the whys and hows of competitive strategy in a changing marketplace.

A successful healthcare campaign will moreover include other initiatives designed to tap into other word-of-mouth networks.

For example, a 10-minute slide presentation on the positioning strategy and campaign will be worn out by the end of the campaign because it will be included and featured at every community education and outreach event during that period of time. It will be shown during every outreach visit to physician offices. It will be shown at every Chamber, Lions, Kiwanis, etc., club meeting of which a system executive or manager is a member.

All the natural, word-of-mouth networks the organization can reach and tap will be made part of the campaign.

2) Women are the primary healthcare decisionmakers.

It is well recognized that women play a dominant role in healthcare purchase decisions. Women purchase and read the healthcare books and magazines. They seek out the information for themselves and their families. Women call the physician referral services. They collect the recommendations from their friends and neighbors.

A recent story illumined this central fact in a slightly different way. A young woman about to give birth to a son was asked by her physician if she wanted them to prepare to circumcise the boy. The doctor explained she didn't do so automatically and that more and more boys were not being circumcised. The young woman asked a few more questions about circumcision, its risks and benefits, and then thought a minute and said, "I don't really know. This is one family health decision I am going to leave to my husband." She informed the baby's father about her conversation with her physician and asked him for his decision—the one family healthcare decision it was surely appropriate for him to make. Her husband thought a minute and said, "Hmm, I don't know either. Let's ask your mom."

Moreover, research again and again confirms that women prefer receiving their healthcare information through direct mail, especially newsletters designed for them, mailed to their homes.

A very important component system of an identity enhancement campaign is a system newsletter designed for and targeted to women. Not only is it a format women appreciate, it is a format that can provide the market a more complete, in-depth understanding than can traditional print and broadcast media. The consumer takes the time to read and understand. It is, moreover, a medium that extends its reach through pass-along to others. Information can be presented that helps consumers understand not only health and illness issues, but also health reform and how to use or not use the resources of the system appropriately.

A system newsletter tells the system story through the medium itself as well as through the message. The fact of the system as the sponsor of the newsletter as opposed to the freestanding hospital, expresses in itself the system identity. Some systems have found such a newsletter a key step in tightening and building more of a sense of systemness among participating member organizations.

The Harris System, for example, in Dallas/Fort Worth selected one women's newsletter for itself and all its member hospitals.

The newsletter comes from the system but with appropriate recognition to the particular member hospital for a given section of the geographic market. Some stories link the market with the system as a whole, others to particular member organizations, such as physician practices, hospitals, home care agencies, etc.

Not only has Harris strengthened its identity as a system, internally and externally, it has also generated a much greater consumer response through its one newsletter for all than it did from the many different newsletters from many different member organizations.

In summary, we can work out of the impossible, but necessary, bind in a Houdini-like fashion if we depend on and follow the method of classic marketing.

We can successfully make an integrated healthcare delivery system a well-understood, preferred option for a given market if we thoroughly understand how the market is making its decisions, reposition the integrated healthcare delivery system in terms of consumer benefits, make those benefits visible, take charge of the brand identity, and break through the clutter with an aggressive integrated communications campaign.

CHAPTER 3

Marketing Authentic Marketing to Healthcare: It's Still the Answer

INTRODUCTION

The healthcare marketing executive's primary challenge is not convincing the marketplace that it should be enamored with a particular healthcare organization, but convincing the healthcare organization that it should be enamored with the marketplace.

The healthcare marketing executive's first responsibility is not marketing the organization to the market, but institutionalizing the marketing concept throughout the healthcare organization. It is the marketing concept or marketing orientation that will become the fertile source of ongoing marketplace solutions and marketplace success. The healthcare marketing executive shouldn't rest until every nook and cranny of the organization has adopted a marketing management philosophy that makes listening to the customer in an in-depth way the first step of service delivery and design. Ironically, the more successful the marketing executive is in changing colleagues within the organization to a marketing philosophy, the more successful the organization will be in the external marketplace. The more thoroughly imbued with a "voice of the customer" attitude the internal stakeholders are—particularly line managers and physicians—the more consistently and irresistibly effective the healthcare organization will be in the marketplace.

It's not enough for a healthcare marketing executive to be a good marketer himself or herself. The test of an effective healthcare marketing executive is whether or not physicians and line managers relish and practice marketing effectively. Most of a healthcare marketing executive's and the healthcare marketing department's time and attention should be oriented towards producing this change in the organization. They need to be deeply inserted into operations for the organization to achieve marketing success. The marketing management set of skills— identifying key target segments, conducting market research, completing marketing plans, doing effective outreach, etc.—all need to be embraced and practiced by the organization as a whole. Not to stay with this bigger vision is to be co-opted into doing peripheral tasks.

This priority is true under all three eras, under the old and new paradigm as well as in the era between the times. It is as true for the healthcare executive of an integrated healthcare delivery system as it is for one working for an HMO, a national nursing home chain, or a hospital.

WHY THE MARKETING OF MARKETING IS THE HEALTHCARE MARKETING EXECUTIVE'S NUMBER-ONE PRIORITY

There are three fundamental reasons why healthcare marketing executives need to make the internal adoption of the marketing concept their highest priority:

1) Healthcare organizations at the outset are not naturally prone to the marketing concept. They are classic expert-oriented organizations.

2) The product "P" of the marketing mix is, in healthcare, not within the province or control of the marketing department. It is the province of the operations staff and physicians. Unless they embrace the marketing concept, the "product" will not be designed to produce customer satisfaction.

3) The product "P" of the marketing mix in healthcare is not a product. A product can be designed once, and if designed well at the outset, incorporating all the features the market is looking for, it can be replicated at will through mass production. The product "P" in healthcare is, on the other hand, a complicated set of services.

Services are people interacting with others to certain ends. By definition, services cannot be mass produced. They are continually dependent on the behavior of people who either do or do not act with the customer mindset.

Healthcare Organizations Are Expert Oriented

Healthcare organizations are classic examples of expert-driven organizations. Healthcare providers think they know their business. They know what's good for the patient. They know what quality is. They know how to evaluate good from bad providers of healthcare. The marketplace doesn't. Their skills and their high technology are what are important. One doesn't listen to the marketplace, one "educates" it.

This cluster of beliefs keeps healthcare organizations from the surprises and successes that come from approaching the customer as the font of marketplace success. The marketing concept reverses the dictates of the expert-driven organization. "Quality is whatever the customer says it is. A good service is defined by the customer in a much broader way than the expert provider defines it. Quality services begin with the customer and their needs, not with the skills and technology of the provider."

It took a very large transformation of cultural attitudes for AT&T to produce the following ad and have its own employees, engineers, and internal constituents believe it and practice it: "Quality is whatever the customer says it is. At AT&T, we think that's the only attitude towards quality that makes sense. All of our technology and skills are at the service of that definition of quality. The customer doesn't know the ins and outs of the technology, but the customer does expect to pick up the phone and have it go through the first time clearly, every time. At AT&T, everything we do is meant to support and deliver on what the customer is expecting."

It's essential that healthcare marketing executives make this their continuing focus, because it takes such great creativity and tenacity to work a cultural transformation in organizations that are as embedded in a reverse posture as are most healthcare organizations.

The Marketer Doesn't Control the Product-or-Place "P"s of the Marketing Mix

An even more fundamental reason for the marketing executive in a healthcare organization to focus on instilling the marketing orientation internally is that in a healthcare organization the marketing executive has no power over the most important "P"s of the marketing mix, namely the Product and Place "P"s. The marketing executive can't control, except indirectly, and can't dictate how services will be designed and delivered. That is the role and responsibility of line managers and physicians. Unless they have the marketing orientation, the products and services will not be designed and delivered in the way the marketplace is expecting.

Imagine, for example, the challenge of marketing an obstetrics service that is still afflicted with the "this is the way we do deliveries here" syndrome. No amount of advertising will produce an uptick in market share until the more basic product and place issues have been addressed by those who can address them, namely physicians and nurses and line managers. Once the voice of the customer has been listened to, heard, and acted upon, the obstetrics service begins to change. One can't market an obstetrics service that pays inadequate attention, for example, to issues of pain management. The availability of 24-hour epidural has become a key issue for a large part of the market. No amount of insistence on physician skills or clinical quality will substitute for the lack of 24-hour epidural. If a significant segment of the market is looking for the services of a midwife, nothing else will satisfy them. If a large part of the market is upset with obstetricians who play "Russian Roulette" with them, who rotate them through their group practice, and can never be clear concerning which physician will be doing the delivery, and if a competitor does it differently, and commits to one or two physicians to be there for the delivery, women will go to that practice rather than to the large group practice. The large group practice that is set up for its own convenience will begin to lose business until it listens to the voice of the consumer. If a large segment has come to think that getting up and moving to a different room for labor, for delivery, and then for recovery is folly, that segment will not be drawn to a facility with old-fashioned labor, delivery, recovery, and post-partum and nursery arrangements.

For all these various segments, the key will be for physicians, nurses, and line managers to make the changes that the market is demanding. The healthcare marketing executive can't make those changes. The healthcare marketing executive's challenge is to have the physicians, nurses, and line managers hear the voice of the consumer in an unvarnished and powerful way, and make sure they follow through on what they have heard.

Eighty percent of the time in healthcare, an organization's lack of success in the marketplace is due to inadequacies of the product and place "P"s of the marketing mix, not to its lack of promotion. Healthcare marketing executives, therefore, need to devote 80 percent of their time to the challenge of getting those inside the organization to make the changes required in the product and place "P"s of the marketing mix.

It was particularly satisfying to hear a physician at a Southern California hospital confess to his colleagues after hearing a series of focus group tapes of women in his marketplace. Focus groups had been conducted with a Japanese segment, a Samoan segment, an Anglo-Saxon upper-class segment, and a Hispanic middle-class segment. Across all four consumer groups, there were some strong common sentiments and some important differentiating aspirations. The physician, who was well and long established in practice, said to his colleagues, "I must admit that for years, nurses and my colleagues and administrators have been telling me that I had to change. Whenever I would hear that from them, I would say to myself, 'No way, I know what's best for my patients. I am the doctor, they are the patient.' I must admit in hearing those focus group tapes and hearing how strong the desire is in women for a range of choices around their childbirth experience, it shook me. I am going to change my ways."

One young physician sitting across from him chafed a bit, knowing that the hospital-sponsored research was producing a converted, potentially more successful competitor to him in practice.

The nurses and the marketing staff around the table kept their smiles in check. They had been planning and facilitating this moment for months. They had hoped that hearing the truth straight from the customer might open the physicians to changing their behavior and make them supportive of the changes the hospital and nurses knew had to be made. They were delighted that it had succeeded. The way was open for them to redesign the physical facility of the obstetrics service and to work with the physicians on collaborative approaches to more adequately satisfy the market.

The healthcare marketing executive trying to produce basic changes in values and orientation needs to have the virtues of the revolutionary. As Camus said, "Patience and irony are the virtues of a revolutionary." Healthcare marketing executives can't look away from this very daunting, at times frustrating, and humanly difficult challenge of engaging and introducing their colleagues across the healthcare organization to the joys of listening to the voice of the customer, and the power of the marketing management discipline.

In some ways, this is no different from any other industry. In other ways, it's much more fundamental and important. This vision of healthcare marketing calls for marketers who are not only technical experts but who are also broad gauge, imaginative leaders.

How long, for example, has it taken for General Motors to get the message about the importance of the voice of the customer? Consider the cover story in *Business Week*, March 21, 1994, titled, "GM's Aurora: Much Is Riding on the Luxury Sedan, and Not Just for Olds." That article explained how important the development of the Aurora is for the future of Oldsmobile and for General Motors and how significantly different its development has been from other product development stories in GM's history. It represents, finally, the embracing by General Motors of the marketing concept. Here is an excerpt:

> At the very least, Aurora is the sign that GM is finally listening to its customers. The number-one car maker had long made a habit of ignoring customer input or delaying market research until the final stages of car development, when it was too late to make changes. By contrast, Aurora's development team consulted extensively with consumer focus groups even before the first designs were drawn. In all, it held 20 so-called clinics nationwide, interviewing more than 4,200 consumers—the biggest such sampling in GM history.
>
> Now the "voice of the consumer" has become GM's new rallying cry. Already the team working on the 1997 Cutlass Supreme has been relying heavily on clinics. GM is re-working and sometimes

even delaying new products that don't please consumers in research groups.

At GM, as in any healthcare organization, the "voice of the consumer" begins to be respected once the organization sees how much more success in the marketplace it enjoys when and if it does pay respect to that voice.

Moreover, there is an intrinsic delight that scientifically oriented professionals take in discoveries that turn the key in the marketplace lock. Good information and good analysis that lead to exciting new insights and effective syntheses are the way of the scientific method and natural to engineers, as in GM, and to physicians, as in a healthcare organization. Once they have been introduced to the power of listening to the consumer, they find the marketing management discipline simpatico with their own psychic and professional bearing and gearing. Instead of equating marketing with promotion, they begin to see it as a method for producing success in the market.

In the story about the development of the Aurora, the process began with good market research. Here is another excerpt from the *Business Week* article:

> In early 1988, Olds gathered owners of European luxury cars, including Mercedes Benz and BMW, in Boston for a clinic. It held similar sessions on the west coast to find out what trendy and import-loving Californians were thinking. Olds' engineer, Douglas L. Stott, says drivers talked about cars that were sporty, with features such as leather seats and wood trim. Performance and quality were a must. They wanted a sophisticated multi-valve engine for smooth acceleration and four-wheel disc brakes. Highest on the list, though, was a nameless characteristic that nearly all the luxury car owners had attempted to describe: something about the solid German cars that inspired confidence and security, gave the vehicles an opulent hush, and isolated drivers from bumps and jolts. Masch and his design team concluded that this sense came from a rock solid body structure.
>
> Working at their facilities in Flint, the engineers went to work testing the rigidity of European imports. In cars, a stiff body produces a high frequency that springs out lower level vibrations such as shakes and rattles. When GM's engineers found the

Mercedes Benz 300 had the highest frequency, at 25 Hz, that became the benchmark. So they began working with design computers and experimenting on plastic scale models and a "mule"— a cobbled together version based on a Sedan DeVille—to find out what it would take to give Aurora the necessary rigid frame.

If it can finally happen at GM after all these decades, it can happen in healthcare organizations if marketing executives find ways to link the voice of the consumer without and the technical experts within.

The Product Is a Service

It is even more important for those at the front line intimately involved in the design and delivery of healthcare services to be imbued with the customer orientation, than it is for workers in product-oriented industries (such as General Motors or Texas Instruments), because services are that much different from products. Products are more readily marketed when they are designed from the ground up to satisfy consumers. The more a product can "sell itself," because it is right on target with what consumers are looking for, the smoother the marketing effort.

Services, however, are triply in need of from-the-ground-up design in terms of customer expectations. Here are the reasons why:

1) There isn't a gap between design, production, and delivery in the case of a service.

A service is produced and delivered at one-and-the-same moment. The ones making the service are, at one and the same time, delivering it.

A product can be designed once and customer satisfaction attributes built into it at the same time. As long as the initial product design is right, all subsequent products, through mass production, can replicate the original design. In the case of a service, however, it has no shelf life. It is totally original each time it is delivered and each time dependent on the attitudes of those delivering it.

2) A service is not just the quality of the human exchange.

A service such as healthcare has much more to it than the moment of human transaction. Any healthcare service is also a whole string of previous human decisions embedded as a set of features and benefits in the moment of encounter. Each of those decisions can be made with the consumer in mind, or they can be made without attention to the consumer. The more thoroughly customer-focused that set of decisions is, the more successful the service.

For example, take the encounter of a patient who has been diagnosed with breast cancer and her physician. From the standpoint of the physician, that encounter is a very complicated set of previous decisions that all converge at the moment of the face-to-face meeting. One physician may come to that moment with a number of convictions and, in effect, decisions already made that are not consumer-friendly. One physician may think that patients need to be sheltered from upsetting information. That physician will be very stingy in the amount of explanation and information provided to the patient. That physician will not even think of inviting the woman's husband for a patient care conference. That physician may have made a decision long before—that he or she will only perform mastectomies or will always make sure that a woman knows clearly what her risks are if there should be a recurrence of breast cancer—which in effect, steers the woman away from any alternative therapy.

Another decision that the physician may have made—which has become calcified into a habit—is the conviction that the quality of his/her surgical skills is the most important issue in the care of the patient. As a result, only in exceptional cases will this particular physician involve adjuvant chemotherapy or even radiation therapy in the treatment of the patient.

What looks like a simple exchange, a service encounter, is actually a very complicated set of previous decisions all converging in the moment of the human encounter. The more all those decisions are made without the customer in mind, the less satisfying will that encounter be. On the other hand, the more the previous decisions have been made with and through the eyes of the customer, the more successful that encounter will be.

Another physician, for example, in that same situation, will be very deeply understanding of the emotions and the fears that the woman is experiencing. He or she will recognize, for example, the woman's fears concerning loss of hair, not being desirable any longer to her husband, and disfigurement. That physician will have followed very closely the research concerning breast conservancy and will not only offer full explanations to the patient, but will also want to make sure that the patient and her husband or loved one understand and follow the facts with the physician so that they, together, can make an informed choice of clinical options. Moreover, that physician will have learned how to perform successful lumpectomies and will be much more ready to involve appropriate medical and radiation oncologists. Moreover, that physician will have involved, from the very first encounter with the patient, the services of a nurse practitioner who can supplement and enhance his or her explanations and ability to be supportive to the patient.

The first challenge for an effective design of a healthcare service is to have all those decisions by the caregivers, embedded in the moment of the encounter, be made or re-made with the customer in mind.

A customer-driven healthcare service is much more than "good bedside manner." As important as the quality of the face-to-face encounter is in the healthcare service, the previous decisions embedded in that encounter are even more important. The more they are all made with the consumer in mind, the more successful the encounter will be in terms of a customer-satisfying performance.

To say that healthcare organizations need to be imbued with the marketing concept is a much, much, more fundamental issue than making the organization customer friendly—although that's part of it. The marketing orientation goes much deeper than mere service excellence. The clinical services themselves need to be designed and delivered from the ground up with the customer in mind. It's not enough to deliver a healthcare service with a smile if the content of the service is anti-consumer.

3) Thirdly, however, it is even more complicated than having care-givers examine, one by one, the bases for their behavior. Even if each caregiver is thoroughly imbued with a customer orientation, that still won't guarantee a customer-satisfying design of a service, because healthcare is actually a cluster of encounters involving many people, functions, and departments.

Healthcare when viewed through the eyes of the customer is more than the moment of interaction with a caregiver. It is actually a whole chain of encounters and impressions.

Reflect, for example, on the following real-life story. A woman with multiple myeloma follows her oncologist from one universi-ty hospital to another where he has accepted an appointment that gives him a higher standing, additional research possibilities, and a larger salary. For three years, they have struggled together with her illness: from acute stages into remission and back into fresh flare-ups. He has monitored, prescribed, explained. She has listened, hoped, coped, and returned. He has read and interpreted the tests, measured and coordinated the medications, observed and discussed their effects, calibrated the adjustments, and set the return appointments. She has felt the effects and side effects of the medication, fought to live a life of independence, struggled to maintain her poise, affections, disposition, and prospects. She has depended on him, respected him, and felt appreciated by him. He recognized the strength of her spirit and tried his best by her.

One day she calls his service in sudden, seizing pain for an appointment. He complies. She arrives at the clinic desk and is told by the receptionist, "I'm sorry, you don't have an appoint-ment," at which she shrinks visibly in a mix of embarrassment and anxiety. She says, "Please check with my doctor—I talked with him on the phone yesterday." The receptionist does so and returns saying, "I am sorry, you do have an appointment." She then waits—an hour, the standard operating procedure—and is then summoned by the nurse to the examining room, where she waits for another hour.

Now, as she is white with pain and just about to leave, her doctor enters the examining room. They have a brief but fairly satisfying conversation. He writes out her medication regimen longhand and explains it to her. As she leaves, she approaches the desk to make her payment. She has called beforehand to arrange to make her payment by check. As she articulates her request to the woman behind the desk, trying to maintain her dignity through the ordeal, she is told, "You cannot do that. Payment for lab and x-ray is additional." She takes time to explain that she has already called and made arrangements to pay the entire bill—lab, x-ray, and physician—with one check. They check further and allow her to pay with one check. She has had the same thing happen every time she has come to that outpatient service.

On the way home from the hospital, she resolves that she is never going back to that hospital. She is returning to the hospital from which her doctor has moved. She understands she would have to laboriously build a relationship with a new oncologist with whatever time is left to her, but decides that is the preferred option to going through the pain, humiliation, and anxiety she has experienced at the second hospital.

What is the product that she is rejecting? Not, in this case, her physician's care. He practices quality medicine even in an expanded sense. He listens, enters into her struggle, recognizes that his service is only part of what she needs to live her life successfully. Nevertheless, despite his excellence, she finds the healthcare wanting.

What is the product or service? The product is actually much more than the interpersonal encounter with the caregiver. It is the *whole experience*—from receptionist through waiting through nurse through physician through transport through billing. That total experience was so negative, so enervating, so different from the warmth and support that she had experienced from the entire staff of the oncology service at the original hospital that it wore her down. Rather than endure it, she left her physician to find healthcare.

To envision, coordinate, and deliver the complicated product health care is, across the whole sequence of the patient pathway in a customer satisfying way, is the central business challenge facing the outpatient service of this university hospital. To break the complicated product healthcare is into its component parts and put it back together again for customer satisfaction is precisely the healthcare marketing challenge. In this situation, it requires a Vice-President of Ambulatory Care, the likely title of the line manager over this disparate group of departments, functions, and moments of the patient pathway, to see his or her role first in terms of his or her marketing management challenge: "design the 'product', i.e., total service, through the eyes of the customer." In turn, the healthcare marketing executive's first obligation is to focus on his or her colleagues in line management, to help them define their roles in terms of marketing, and to give them all the help they need to successfully carry out *their* marketing challenges.

Given the range of businesses under a healthcare organization's umbrella and the range of the departments, functions, and people involved, the healthcare marketing executive's more than full-time challenge is to—might and main—get all those functions and departments—working through existing structures and systems—to embrace the marketing concept.

THE INTERNAL CHALLENGE REMAINS THE CENTRAL CHALLENGE IN THE NEW PARADIGM AND BETWEEN THE TIMES

This vision of healthcare marketing that gives priority attention to marketing to internal constituents is true not just for those involved in healthcare delivery organizations such as hospitals, clinics, home-care agencies, and nursing homes. It is just as true, and perhaps even more so, for healthcare marketing executives working with **integrated health-care delivery systems** and with **health maintenance organizations.** The temptation of a healthcare marketing executive at a hospital system level or working for an integrated healthcare delivery system is to become too removed from the way the marketplace actually works. The temptation is to be subsumed into the world of big, strategic decisions to the neglect of transforming the organization for marketplace success.

Take, for example, the vice-president of marketing at a major integrated healthcare delivery system in the Midwest, who successfully resisted that temptation and kept true to the vision of "first make the changes inside."

From the moment he took the job, he identified the major weakness of the system, the variable that would either make or break its success over time: lack of access to the system's primary-care physicians. It was hard to get appointments, patients had long waits after they arrived, and caregivers acted rushed and abrupt.

Consistently over the course of two years, he has used all his skills and power to work a transformation of that key variable in the operating units.

The system employs hundreds of physicians in well-distributed clinics throughout a geographic region. That is both its strength and its potential vulnerability because the physicians have had no more room for patients. Current members of affiliated HMOs are disenchanted with the level of services that they receive from these physician clinics. The system can't attract more business to itself because of the difficulties of getting appointments with the primary-care physicians.

This vice-president of marketing has hundreds of requests and bids for his time and his staff's time and resources: product line campaigns, hospital promotions, public relations events, new market feasibility analyses, new opportunities for mergers and acquisitions, patient satisfaction systems within the system-owned hospitals, senior programs, women's health initiatives, etc. With all the competing bids for his time and attention, he has never lost sight of this central issue at the clinic level.

Some told him that it was an intractable problem that could never be fixed. The physicians would never change their behaviors. They could not be made to work harder. He should turn his attention to other areas where he could have more influence. He refused, however, to turn away from what he saw was the fundamental flaw of the system's "product."

He used all four sources of power available to him to work with others to eventually change the situation. Those sources are as follows:

1) He used market research.

Consumer focus groups confirmed existing and potential patients' frustrations. By sharing these testimonials in an unvarnished way with physician and clinic leadership, he began to get them to see the issue through the eyes of the customer. Once the physicians and clinic management were confronted with the information, they were embarrassed and were not as comfortable with "business as usual" and with structuring physicians' schedules around the convenience of the physicians.

2) He used the tools of customer flow analysis.

They realized that the problem of access was not as much a problem of demand, as much as it was a problem of management of supply. It was not really an insufficient number of physicians, nor was it a question of too many requests for service. It was a question of the way the supply of physicians was being managed. For example, once physicians went to lunch together in the middle of the day, it was difficult to get back on a rational schedule for patients. Moreover, there were clear peaks and valleys of customer demand and requests. Those factors had not been factored into the scheduling of physicians' time. This information began to be used to develop schedules around the peaks and valleys.

3) He used the tools of peer pressure and peer modeling.

As some clinics began to reorganize themselves into panels of patients and began to more successfully handle their panels of patients, as they began to staff themselves more rationally around the graphed patterns of patient demand, their patient satisfaction ratings began to edge upwards. These clinics began to be models of behavior for others. Others began to see that there was no real rational reason for them to be receiving negative patient satisfaction scores on the grounds of poor access.

4) He used the power of organizational politics and top-down pressures.

Working with the physician and administrative leadership at the executive level, they all began to see the importance of holding physicians accountable for a targeted number of clinical hours of performance. No one had ever really held physicians to their standards. Moreover, they developed new incentive programs for physicians who worked harder and reduced rewards for those who fell below the established criteria of 35 hours a week of clinical contact time.

For the first time in a long time, the whole system begins to see that it can be attracting more volume. Problems of access begin to ease, and the organization again takes on an entrepreneurial, hungry, formidable air as it goes after additional marketshare on both its fee-for-service and covered-lives fronts—the old and the new paradigms.

That marketing executive exemplifies the central tenet of this chapter. The healthcare marketing executive's primary responsibility is infusing a marketing orientation into the entire organization.

Healthcare marketing executives working for HMOs are recognizing the same priority. Before tackling the marketplace, one has to tackle one's own organization. While trying to market the organization to the marketplace, one has to spend as much time or more time marketing marketing to the organization. In a *Modern Healthcare* story of November 7, 1994, Mary Chris Jaklevic presents the recent experience of Kaiser Permanente in San Diego. The article begins:

> Three years ago, after a rapid spurt of growth, Kaiser Permanente in San Diego found itself with an embarrassing problem: bad service. In non-urgent cases, patients frequently had to wait five weeks to see a specialist at the HMO. Elective surgery could take two or three months to schedule.

As many new enrollees as Kaiser succeeded in signing up each year, just as many were going out the back door each year because of dissatisfaction. The article continues, "Among enrollees who left, poor service and lack of appointment access were cited three times as often as complaints about cost, location or coverage."

The leadership of the organization recognized that they needed to bring to the table the strong voice of the customer in order to produce a turnaround internally. The article continues:

> "My task as the marketing manager was to bring the marketplace to Kaiser," said Dennis Humberstrom, Kaiser's district manager.
>
> "Employee benefits managers were invited to meet with Kaiser's medical director, hospital administrator and chiefs of service. Benefits managers asked why they shouldn't switch to cheaper plans to promise better access. It was the first time providers had heard directly from purchasers. It made a huge difference," Mr. Humberstrom said.
>
> Thus began a slow process of change. The employer advisory council helped develop access standards, including specialty appointments within two weeks 80 percent of the time, Sunday

appointments for primary care, and operating room access for elective surgery within four weeks 80 percent of the time.

Kaiser's 478 physicians and 4,700 non-physician staff members responded with a host of low cost innovations, such as direct booking for specialty appointments at primary-care offices, more open appointment times, and follow-up visits by telephone or by primary-care physicians rather than specialists.

In time, most targets were met . . . Kaiser's marketshare has held steady since.

Healthcare marketing executives across the healthcare industry have the same challenge. Many are effective marketers in their own right. The marketing challenge they face is the most daunting of all, marketing marketing to those inside their organizations. The test of a good marketing executive is not that *they* can do marketing effectively, but whether or not their colleagues, especially line managers, physicians, and operations staff take to and learn how to practice effective marketing.

How to Instill the Marketing Orientation into a Healthcare Organization

The four most powerful strategies for instilling a marketing orientation throughout a healthcare organization are:

1) Use qualitative market research.

2) Make marketing the subject of a management system.

3) Provide simple to use formats to operating unit managers to develop their own marketing plans.

4) Utilize the bureaucracy and the existing organizational lines of power to force the issue of key changes in service design.

All four of these tools and strategies are best first demonstrated in numerous settings, and then work most powerfully when they are institutionalized, made into organizational expectations and weaved into the day-to-day rhythm of the life of the organization.

Strategy #1: Demonstrate, codify, and then institutionalize market research as the font of service design and delivery

The most powerful ally in converting a product-driven or expert-driven organization to a marketing concept is good market research, well utilized. When healthcare executives, board members, physicians, and line managers experience how rich the insights that come from good market research are; how clearly good market research can point out the path to differential advantage; and how powerful strategies that emerge from good market research are, the organization begins in a new way to have a respect for the voice of the consumer.

When an organization begins to consistently include market research at the front end of its planning; makes it a requirement for all important decisions; and a requirement for all attempts to refashion or improve the quality of services, then the organization takes a step towards being market oriented.

When, in addition, market research becomes part of the ongoing rhythm of the way operating units are managed from day to day; is always given priority in annual budgets; and the results are studied carefully and shared widely within an organization, then the organization is indeed well on its way to becoming market driven.

The healthcare marketing executive, therefore, proceeds in three stages with good market research: first, **demonstrate**; second, **codify**; third, **institutionalize**.

In the first stage, when first taking on the responsibility for marketing or when finally given a free hand to practice effective marketing, the healthcare executive makes sure that he or she has enough resources in his or her own budget to be able to provide good marketing research as often as possible to the organization. In this stage, the healthcare marketer demonstrates good market research, provides it, and insists on it at every opportunity.

In the second stage, once the executive team begins to see the ongoing critical value of good market research, the marketing executive prompts the executive team to make market research a normative expectation in a range of different settings. For example, "In order for a budget to go forward to the board suggesting an expansion of a service, a section documenting the market research basis for the projected volume should always accompany the budget and request for capital." In this second stage, the spirit begins to be codified. Good examples that are designed to be contagious evolve into clearer organizational expectations and protocols.

In the third stage, market research is woven into the fabric of the way the organization is managed daily. In the final stage of maturity, the organization consistently makes the voice of the consumer the touchstone of decisionmaking, evaluation, and benchmarking. Operating units are expected to budget for and regularly conduct market research studies—not just when embarking on new services, but also when deciding how to improve current ones.

The healthcare marketing executive knows that it's not good enough for marketers to appreciate and be able to use good market research. The organization will not be powerfully market oriented until managers, physicians, and staff members across the organization begin to relish, appreciate, and use market research.

The kind of market research that is most useful for these purposes is not typically quantitative market research. There is frequently some confusion over when to use quantitative market research in the form of surveys and when to use "softer" market research, such as focus groups and in-depth personal interviews. Most often, the challenge for marketing in its intersection with physicians and line managers is to help them *improve* their services, to make the design and delivery of a particular service *better*. The kind of information that yields insights into how to improve a service is in-depth, qualitative information. That information comes from deep probing of people's desires, frustrations, and expectations. A survey instrument is not the appropriate vehicle for developing this kind of information. A survey instrument is best for determining how many people feel a certain way or how large a given market is. Even using open-ended questions in a quantitative survey, while instinctively in the right direction, never quite gets at the information desired. In order to get the information into a computer, the hundreds of different responses to an open-ended question are lumped and homogenized.

Instead, it makes sense to utilize the tools of qualitative market research when desiring in-depth insights into how to make a program or service more responsive to consumer expectations. Those tools, as most healthcare marketing professionals know, are the tools of focus groups and in-depth personal interviews.

Focus Groups Are Golden Tools for Transforming the Culture.

The most valuable kind of market research for working this transformation is not quantitative research or survey research—although such research plays an important contributing role—the most valuable type of research for stimulating behavior change and respect for the consumer is in-depth, qualitative market research. And the technique of qualitative research that is the most valuable is focus group research.

Focus groups are in-depth sessions with a randomly selected target market segment of 10 to 12 members, lasting some two hours, concerning a specific subject matter; conducted by a qualified moderator following a topical guide; and probing the participants' thoughts, feelings, motivations, and expectations. A topical guide is an outline developed by leadership of all the most important issues and concerns that leadership wants to hear about from the marketplace.

Good focus groups convene a homogeneous group of target market members (primary-care physicians aren't mixed with surgeons; former patients aren't mixed with nonpatients; etc.). This allows an in-depth discussion in which participants in the focus group stimulate one another, bounce off one another, and eventually get to their deeper levels of motivation and expression. A good focus group is almost impossible to shut off. Because knowledgeable consumers have been recruited concerning the topic at issue, and they begin to spark one another's ideas and deeper emotions, it is a very rich and rewarding experience for those who participate.

Qualitative, in-depth insights are what are needed in most healthcare management decision settings. In order to *improve* a service, which is typically the most important marketing issue, leadership needs in-depth information, not the results of survey research. Survey research says *how many* people feel a certain way; it doesn't get at *how* people feel. Most of the time, the results of qualitative research stand on their own. The insights are garnered and changes are made. At other times, it is important to follow up the qualitative research with quantitative research to make sure that the insights coming out of the focus group of 10 to 12 participants—or more typically a series of focus groups—really does represent the marketplace as a whole. The results of qualitative research are not projectable to the population. That, however, is not typically the purpose of qualitative research. Typically, the question that is being asked of the market is not how many people think a certain way. The question is what do people think.

Good qualitative research is valuable in at least five different ways. It alerts leaders how:

1) to avoid major pitfalls and potential gaffes;

2) to reconfigure services so that they are more aligned with what the marketplace is seeking;

3) to prioritize particular strategies and tactics;

4) to prompt behavior changes on the part of the providers; and

5) to see the opportunities in the marketplace, and therefore, bring diverse groups together behind marketplace opportunities.

Avoid major pitfalls and potential gaffes.

Whenever an operating unit is considering a major innovation or departure from business as usual, it makes sense to test the suggested "improvements" with the marketplace to garner its reaction and guidance.

Not long ago, a major medical center was planning a new cancer center and was about to initiate construction. Physician and management leadership was confident that the new design of the cancer center would be much superior to the center that patients had utilized in the past. Leadership decided to test the program design as well as a number of other hypotheses and issues with current and former patients of their center.

Focus group participants were delighted that all the outpatient cancer services would now be centralized at one location with more accessible parking. A number of major concerns, however, surfaced in both focus groups conducted with current and former patients. One, participants were very upset at the area of separate waiting rooms for gowned patients and their friends or relatives, and the separate waiting rooms for men and women in the radiation therapy area. The separate waiting area for family/friends and gowned patients was perceived as diminishing the sense of community and support they seek while undergoing treatment. A range of quotes illustrates how strongly patients felt about this issue and how convincing their testimony was to physician and management leadership.

"It is better to bring your friends in with you." (group 1)

"Yes, you don't want to be alone. You'd rather have them there." (group 1)

"I think you need the support of your family and your friends during this time." (group 1)

"To seclude them is really stupid." (group 1)

"I think they should have a dressing room and from there, you go to a waiting area." (group 2)

"I have very strong feeling about that. You depend on your family to get through this and you don't want them in the other room." (group 1)

Moreover, participants absolutely and intensely disliked the idea of having separate waiting areas for men and women once gowned. Many bring a spouse or other support person with them, and want to wait with that person. They appreciate and look forward to the camaraderie of sharing their experiences with a consistent group of other patients, regardless of gender.

"That stinks." (group 1)

"I also don't like this male/female deal. I mean the dressing rooms are okay —" (group 1)

"I don't see the need for a sexual differentiation. Because you talk to the people that you're waiting with." (group 1)

"My husband sat beside me the whole time." (group 1)

"A problem with separate rooms would be that oftentimes my husband comes with me. I'm too sick to come myself. So where would the two of us go?" (group 2)

Moreover, the participants suggested a much closer relationship between the treatment areas, the exam rooms, and the reception area.

The basic design of the center was reviewed and redone. By testing the design on knowledgeable customers, some serious problems with the design were avoided.

Illustrate how to provide differential advantages in services.

In this same example of the proposed new outpatient cancer center, participants indicated that they would like to see clearly designated refreshment areas stocked with a variety of beverages and light, healthy snacks that reflected the types of dietary limitations of many cancer patients.

They compared experiences at different centers.

"My last two weeks of radiation, I had to take it at "X" Medical Center, because all the machines here had broke. Their cancer center makes this place look, you know. It was all bright and new and cheery. It was on the main floor, it wasn't in the basement . . . it was all bright. You walked in and they had food . . . some days they had cheesecake and some days they had fruit . . . some days they had bread and muffins. It was different every day. It was very spread out. It wasn't real cramped like it is downstairs. What made that miserable two weeks very doable is that it wasn't in the basement. It was open and windows and they had valet parking." (group 1)

"I always grab a can of pop when I leave the office. I'll take a bottle of juice and I think that's great. I really like that. But if I could pick up an apple, I don't think I'd mind if I had to pay for it." (group 1)

"Especially fresh fruits and good fruits. Fruits like kiwis and stuff like that." (group 2)

Physician and management leadership could see that the quality of the environment, in particular, a refreshment center, could be a "cue to quality" that was meaningful to patients. Kiwi fruit isn't important in and of itself, but in this competitive situation, it serves as the final, fine touch of customer-sensitive treatment.

Moreover, patients pointed the way to an even more fundamental differentiating feature for their cancer service—a focus on wholistic care.

"I really like our doctors, the practice, the care and the nurses, but I would like to see comprehensive care for the whole body . . . that means not only treating the disease, trying to kill it, but also trying to boost your immune system by proper diet and nutrition. Exercise. Vitamin therapy . . . also for your mind and spirit. Counseling. I would like to see it all in one area." (group 1)

"I do that on my own and I don't know what I'm doing." (group 1)

"So you don't have to go see the nutritionist somewhere else." (group 1)

"Diet was never mentioned when I was having chemo and radiation." (group 2)

"They just told you what you shouldn't eat." (group 2)

For a cancer center set up according to very traditional clinical lines, it was apparent that patients were defining cancer treatment much more broadly. A focus on the whole body, and the spirit, was not perceived as out of the mainstream of medicine, but responsive and exactly on target to what they were experiencing from day to day.

Physician and management leadership rethought and reconfigured the constellation of services that would be provided in the new cancer center. They added the integrated services of nutritionists, support groups, and counseling. They also added music therapy to their array of services and a much closer link with the pastoral care program.

Reprioritize particular strategies and tactics.

At times, healthcare professionals listening to the marketplace find their preconceptions shaken and their sense of priorities questioned.

A series of focus groups conducted with senior citizens in an Ohio city, for example, testing proposed initiatives from the healthcare organization towards the senior market, turned the providers' priorities upside down. Going into the focus groups, the moderator was to test in order of importance a series of services and/or initiatives aimed at responding to seniors' needs. The first item listed was a geriatric assessment center. The second was an Alzheimer's program. The third was a geropsych program. The fourth was a senior wellness center, etc. Way down at the bottom of the list came a senior membership program, dismissed by the professionals as not having substance.

The focus group participants were clear that the healthcare organization would do them the most benefit if they initiated a senior membership program that promised help with Medicare paperwork. Frustrations with Medicare paperwork were so high and so intensely felt by the market that the first healthcare organization to offer such assistance would shift their loyalties.

A geriatric assessment center was listed as least important and rated the lowest in terms of their perceived needs.

Prompt behavior change on the part of providers.

One of the challenges in healthcare is getting colleagues to see what the market is saying. Unless a whole group of providers can be convinced that the marketplace is wanting change, it is not likely that the provider community will change.

A university hospital on the East Coast had a very surprising set of discoveries emerge from their focus groups with referring physicians. They were testing various improvements they were planning in their cancer program.

The participants in the focus groups were very clear that the first and most important improvement that needed to be made was improving the internal relationships between the head of radiation oncology and the head of medical oncology.

> "Oncology—the best way to describe it is fire and ice. Dr. X, the head of Radiation Oncology, is ice and Dr. Y, the head of Medical Oncology, is fire. They just don't get along." (group 1)

Another physician referred to the strife that was obvious to referring physicians.

> "It's sort of a city-wide joke that there are always battles going on there." (group 2)

> "This politics business doesn't look nice at all; but I really don't know that you mean the patient is getting the wrong care because of this." (group 1)

> "If you send someone to a medical oncologist and the patient needs radiation therapy and the two groups never talk to each other— that's not the way to treat a patient." (group 1)

> "There are many other choices in town. When medical oncology and radiation therapists don't talk to each other, like each other, work with each other well, there's no point in sending someone there." (group 2)

Physician and administrative leadership were chastened to know that the conflicts internally were so well known in the general community and were obviously affecting referral decisions. Even the two physicians at issue, while at first very upset with the findings of the market research, nonetheless committed to change their behavior and to begin cooperating with one another.

Clinical professionals, especially physicians, may not see the importance of changing behavior just because nurses or administrators or even their own colleagues tell them that behavior change is warranted. When, however, their customers on whom they depend for a living indicate that they should be changing their behaviors, it has an altogether greater power of persuasion.

Qualitative market research has a self-authenticating ring to it. Witnessing customers' reactions and testimony in person, behind a two-way mirror, or even watching it on a videotape or listening to an audiotape has a power that no survey research or summary documentation can have. The voice of the customer speaks in his or her own words.

Point out opportunities in the marketplace, and therefore, bring diverse groups together.

A few years ago, the country's most profitable nursing home chain conducted a series of focus groups with primary-care physicians, selected specialists, and case managers of insurance companies to assess their interest in subacute services. They expressed such a vibrant interest in the subacute care option that the nursing home chain was able to get its whole executive team united behind an aggressive, capital-intensive initiative in this direction. They are now the leading company in subacute care, as well as being the most profitable of all national nursing home chains.

A medical center with a neurosciences institute that was having trouble bringing its neurologists and neurosurgeons together, began to be galvanized once the physicians reviewed the market research concerning the potential for a collaborative program in the treatment and management of stroke patients. The research was conducted with paramedics and representative pre-hospital providers of care such as police and fire departments. Additional focus groups were conducted with primary-care physicians. All testified to the lack of a center in the marketplace that specialized in the handling of stroke patients. There were plenty of rehabilitation programs treating stroke after the acute phase, but no place that encouraged the early treatment of stroke as "a brain attack" similar to the approach taken with heart attacks.

In order to put together a strong and well-regarded program and center for stroke, neurologists, neurosurgeons, internists, and emergency room physician, all begin to plan together.

Finding opportunities in the marketplace that promise a bigger pie for all is the surest method for overcoming traditional turf battles. If all participants can see that there will be more for them if they cooperate than if they go it alone, they are more likely to cooperate.

A successful marketing power will move past using good marketing research to institutionalizing its use.

A first-rate example of an organization that has evolved into this third stage of maturity is Lutheran General HealthSystem in Park Ridge, Ill. At this point in its history, it is a normal and natural way of doing business for line managers and physicians to consistently, if not annually, conduct qualitative market research studies to reinvigorate their understanding of their customers and/or fine tune their services to be even more successful in the marketplace. Within the last year, for example, this is a sample listing of constituents with whom the Medical Center has conducted in-depth research:

- oncology patients
- rehabilitation patients and caregivers
- cervical cancer patients
- independent living center residents
- long-term care residents' caregivers and referral sources

All across the health system, internal constituents have become aware of and convinced of the ongoing value of good market research. As that has developed, the organization has become more and more customer oriented and successful in the marketplace.

In sum, there is no ally for converting an organization to a marketing mindset quite as powerful as excellent, insightful qualitative market research. Helping physicians and line managers avoid problems, improve services, show differential advantage, and attract market share makes them want more of the same. Once they have learned the charm and appeal of listening to the marketplace, they find it hard to get enough.

The healthcare marketing executive, therefore, first demonstrates and ignites a spark, then codifies the enthusiasm for good market research, and finally institutionalizes it so that it is an organizational value and habit.

Note: Some may have initial misgivings at the thought of "institutionalizing" market research, i.e., making it an ongoing activity of the multiple operating units within a healthcare organization, and including it in the budgets of the operating units. The first misgiving may be around how to coordinate a welter of market research studies and how to assure a high level of quality. The second misgiving may be around expense.

In response to the first misgiving, a healthcare organization that values market research does not have to end up fragmentary in its approach to conducting market research. The healthcare marketing executive and his or her marketing department will serve as the ongoing coordinator of a range of market research studies. The professional marketer will best be able to find the right vendors of market research, make sure that the methodology of the studies is quality, and either conduct the studies or make sure that vendors conduct the studies in a first-rate fashion. It is important to reiterate that the more market research that is done, the better. A healthcare organization of any size typically has so many lines of business under its umbrella, that multiple market research studies are more than warranted in a given year. The professional marketing department serves as the conduit and the provider of professional assistance, but does not strangle the burgeoning interest in market research all across the organization. The healthcare marketing executive and the professional marketers will be overjoyed at seeing many blossoms bloom.

The second misgiving relating to expense is best answered in terms of return on investment thinking. All the examples used in this chapter have powerful return on investment implications. Costly mistakes avoided, differential advantage achieved, new markets discovered, and market share gains secured are what come out of good market research. An industry that is spending five percent of gross revenue on information systems that serve mainly to simply gauge how the organization is performing should definitely devote resources to making sure the organization performs more successfully. Most of the huge expenditure annually on information only tracks an organization's internal performance. Much more valuable is information about the external customer that prompts improved performance.

A second part of the answer, however, relates to the expense of actually conducting first-rate qualitative market research. A typical focus group conducted by a professional research compny—including the costs of the expense of recruiting the focus group in a way that doesn't produce bias—conducting the focus group in a setting that doesn't produce bias, and providing incentives to participants, runs between $3,000 and $4,000. (Incentives for physician participation today range from $100 to $200. Incentives to consumers for participating range from $30 to $50 per participant.) The organization can break out the costs of a focus group and take on parts of the overall project internally, and therefore, save on the overall cost of $3,000 to $4,000 per focus group.

Figure 3-1 shows that a focus group budget may be broken out into the following nine components:

The $3,000 to $4,000 expense will be lower, for example, if the transcripts are done internally; or only a top-line brief report and recommendations is requested; or a personal presentation by the outside market research consultant is not required; or a hotel meeting room is used instead of a dedicated focus group facility that allows for direct client observation through a one-way mirror.

Also note that there are economies to conducting focus groups in multiples. Fixed costs such as development of the discussion guide and report preparation can be spread across multiple groups. Facility rental per group often is decreased if multiple groups are conducted "back-to-back" in the same evening.

Given the suggestions concerning how to conduct qualitative research efficiently—if not on a shoestring—it is important to reiterate once again that there are very few expenditures that produce as great a return, and very few investments of time, energy, and resources that produce such a double-barreled impact of giving an operating unit an insight into how to conduct business better, and at the same time contributing to the turn of the entire organization to a marketing consciousness.

Figure 3-1: Typical Focus Group Budget Categories

Design of the study and development of a topical guide; coordinate recruitment and arrangements	$800–$1,000	Professional consulting time
Recruitment of each focus group	$600–$900	A specialized professional service
Incentives (allow 12 per group)	$400–$600 (consumers) $1,000–$2,000 (physicians)	
Facility rental, audiotaping, and participant and observer needs	$500–$800	Range depends on facility
The actual conducting of the focus group	$250–$300	Professional consulting time
Video recording of the focus group (optional: stationary or manned)	$125–$500 per group	Tech time and materials
Transcript of each focus group	$150–$200	Typist time
A written report on the results of the focus group that identifies the major themes and findings, weaves in helpful quotes to illustrate the findings, and an analysis and set of recommendations	$1,000–$2,000	Professional consulting time
A presentation of the focus group report to a leadership team	$250–$300	Professional consulting time

Quantitative Attitude Research as Another Important Ally.

Another important set of data for a healthcare organization is how it is perceived by its key constituents.

For a managed-care company, it is critical for success to monitor the degree in which it is perceived by area physicians as a "1-800-DENY" type managed-care organization. It is difficult to recruit the right kind of physicians to participate in a particular PPO or HMO if the HMO or PPO has the reputation in the marketplace for withholding care from patients as its financial strategy.

It is well-known to healthcare provider systems and hospitals that the way they are perceived by the general public and employers is important for their long-range success. Good community attitude, employer attitude, physician attitude, and employee attitude research provides baseline measures against which to set marketing objectives and measure progress. Moreover, such objective information widely shared can serve as a goad to the entire organization. Coordinated efforts to improve customer perceptions are better understood and supported if internal constituents know the competitive perception data that prompt and warrant the initiatives.

If an organization is perceived as inferior to competitors by key constituents, it is very important for the whole internal family to see and understand that information. It is much easier to generate a united effort to achieve certain progress towards objectives if all know what the stakes are, what the starting points are, and are able to track progress together as the organization changes the market's perceptions.

Moreover, such attitudinal research gives an organization the ability to notch progress and to establish an ongoing rhythm of celebration of achievement. In this way, it helps build a common culture that starts with, continues to pay attention to, and in some ways, ends with how the customer perceives the organization. As such, it facilitates the shift to the marketing concept.

This type of quantitative perceptual data builds a customer consciousness **from the top down**—providing those down through the organization an understanding of how the organization as a whole is perceived. It works well with qualitative research—which builds a customer consciousness in the innards of the organization and builds a customer consciousness **from the bottom up**—as operating unit after operating unit conducts and benefits from its own in-depth qualitative market research studies.

In summary, the healthcare marketing executive desiring to work a cultural change in his or her healthcare organization finds market research to be a powerful tool for working that transition. It serves, as it has in other industries, as the link between the customer without and the experts within, it turns out that market research gives physicians and other caregivers a way to get inside their management challenges that is quite familiar and comfortable to them from clinical situations. Just as physicians labor on the front end to get a comprehensive, in-depth understanding of a patient's situation in order to make a diagnosis and a subsequent prescription and care plan; so also on the management side of their responsibilities, market research provides the comprehensive picture of the marketplace and its needs and wants, which: justifies, and leads to an accurate prescription and path of action. As diagnosis drives treatment clinically, so market research drives strategy in the business setting. As such, it is a natural, familiar dynamic for clinicians, and one which—once they are exposed to it—they find very congenial.

Strategy #2: Imitate how finance has worked a cultural change in healthcare organizations—make marketing the subject of a management system

The second important strategy for a healthcare marketing executive to utilize in turning a healthcare organization on to the marketing concept is to follow the lead of another staff-to-line function that has worked such a cultural transformation before marketing, namely the finance function.

Finance evidences seven attributes that have made it a discipline that is thoroughly integrated into the fabric of healthcare organizations. They are worth emulating.

1) At this point in history, most healthcare organizations are thoroughly versed in the business discipline of finance. Financial management is a **cultural value** in healthcare organizations. It is assumed that healthcare organizations should be responsibly managed from the standpoint of its use of resources and capital. It is assumed in this point in history, that even a not-for-profit healthcare organization should produce a return on its investment and maintain profitability.

   Apparently, this was not always so. Healthcare organizations began to develop their financial management capabilities in a major way in the mid-'60s—prompted by the passage of Medicare.

2) Today, as it is in most other industries, a "Chief Financial Officer" is the title in a healthcare organization for the **staff person who symbolizes, nurtures, and leads the organization** in terms of its fiscal duties and activities.

   This title has steadily evolved from the early years when the key finance person was called "Accountant," then "Patient Accounts Manager," "Controller," "Director of Finance," "Vice-President of Finance," and finally "C.F.O."—reflecting the evolution, clarification, and expansion of the role.

3) Finance today is woven into the day-to-day business dealings of a successful healthcare organization. It is the **subject of a management system**. Everyone knows when the budgets are due. The budget-setting rhythm annually involves operating units, senior management, and the board in an iterative process.

4) Managers across and down a healthcare organization are **evaluated** at this point in time, partially in terms of their shouldering of financial management responsibilities. Achieving productivity targets and managing against a budget are givens of today's healthcare organizations.

5) Finance provides managers down and across the organization with the **basic tools** that they need to perform *their* financial management roles. Budget packages with forms and instructions are handed out annually. Budgeting and financial management workshops are conducted by finance for individual operating unit managers. Hands-on assistance is provided by finance staff to the operating unit managers.

6) **Information systems** are developed and implemented so that timely, accurate, and helpful financial management information is made available to the operating units. With this information they are able to track progress, make mid-course corrections, and carry out successfully their financial management responsibilities.

7) An **ongoing rhythm of evaluation** is built into the annual calendar of the organization to track progress towards financial management objectives. From the board on down, a first item on a meeting agenda is how the organization as a whole, individual operating units, etc., are performing vis-à-vis their financial targets. Quarterly review is standard.

Finance symbolizes financial management, but the whole organization knows that finance doesn't produce the bottom line, or on a day-to-day basis, manage the whole organization. Finance is a classic staff-to-line function providing supportive services, education, tools, and management systems that others use to carry out their responsibilities. Any effective chief financial officer in a healthcare organization when asked, "Do you produce the bottom line?" will answer, "I'm on for reporting it. My colleagues in operations/line management produce the bottom line."

The analogy between the way finance has been thoroughly integrated into healthcare organizations and marketing's course of action is one to one. Figure 3-2 demonstrates that graphically.

Figure 3-2: Finance as Marketing's Model for Working a Change in the Culture of a Healthcare Organization

	FINANCE	MARKETING
Iterative annual process	Time each year when budgets are due	Time each year when the marketing plans are due
Tools for helping line managers	• Budget development package: forms, instructions	• Marketing plan development package: forms and instruction
	• Budgeting and financial management workshops	• Marketing management workshops
	• Hands-on assistance	• Hands-on assistance
Performance evaluation	Financial objectives used in evaluation of performance	Business Development performance used in evaluating managers
	• Budget measures	• Volume
	• Productivity measures	• Satisfaction
Signs of sophistication	Managers know their fixed and variable costs	Managers know how to identify lush, underserved segments
Information provided	Timely financial information	Timely marketing information
Regular review by Senior Management and Board	Quarterly review of progress towards financial objectives	Quarterly review of progress towards business development objectives
Specialized contributions	Manage arbitrage, conduct financial modeling, etc.	Manage market research, ad campaigns, media relations, etc.

Comparisons Between Finance and Marketing.

- Just as finance, fiscal responsibility, and achieving a bottom line are strong cultural values within a healthcare organization, the advent of effective marketing leadership, the voice of the consumer, the importance of the customer as the source of program design and delivery, and the focus on customer satisfaction as the key variable in an organization's success also are enmeshed in the organization as cultural values.

- Just as the organization has a chief financial officer who symbolizes and stands for effective financial management, so also the organization has a chief marketing officer or healthcare marketing executive who stands for and helps the organization become a powerful marketing force. However, the healthcare marketing executive doesn't perform all facets of marketing in lieu of the operating managers.

For example, one hospital in North Carolina has an ongoing, friendly debate and rivalry between the vice-president of finance who is known as "Suckee Ho" among his colleagues in administration, and the vice-president of marketing who is known as "Ferti Gro." Each executive is well thought of by his peers and valued by the chief executive officer. The vice-president of finance is known as one who is always saying, "Suck in and hold on." The way to success in the marketplace according to him is strong financial controls and a lean operating budget. Supplementing this point of view is the vice-president of marketing who is always insisting and trying to show how "this business can be grown" and developed. Both voices are valued by the chief executive officer. Together they make for **the right combination of energies—** effective control and responsible use of resources, together with a focus on the marketplace, a going after competitive advantage, and an organization that is not just lean and mean but also robust and growing.

- Marketing will successfully follow in the footsteps of finance once the healthcare marketing executive has made marketing the subject of a marketing management system, just as finance is the subject of a financial management system. This means that the organization will have cleared a time for marketing management just as it has cleared a time for financial management.

Nothing happens within a healthcare organization unless it is put on the organization's calendar. That's why it has been so important to have a preestablished calendar for the development of the budget. Unless the organization is alerted early to when the operating units need to have their budgets completed, and when senior management needs to complete the overall budget, it will not be done in a timely fashion from year to year. The calendar pivot point in most healthcare organizations is the board meeting at which the budget will finally be approved.

Marketing also is not **spread through the organization as a management discipline** until the calendar is established that specifies when individual operating units' marketing plans are due and when senior management will have made its selection of the organization's priority marketing objectives for the year. Marketing becomes the subject of a management system once it is integrated into the annual calendar. A pivot point in the organization's annual life is—once marketing is perceived as the integrating management discipline—when the board reviews and approves the strategic marketing plan for the organization. In fact, that decision begins to influence and drive the budget rather than the other way around.

• Just as finance enables the operating managers and physicians within the healthcare organization to perform their financial management responsibilities by first providing them with tools and instructions for completing a budget, so also the healthcare marketing executive facilitates operating unit managers and physicians taking on their marketing management responsibilities by providing them with **marketing plan formats and instructions.** Just as finance works with managers to help them develop their skills by providing budgeting and financial management workshops, so also the healthcare marketing executive helps operating unit managers and physicians learn the marketing management discipline by providing them with marketing management workshops. Just as finance provides hands-on assistance during the period when managers are completing their budgets, so also marketing staff members provide hands-on, ongoing assistance to managers as they complete their marketing plans in an annual fashion.

• Just as financial objectives such as budget performance and productivity measures are used in evaluating managers and that information is integrated into their overall performance evaluation, so also **managers are evaluated,** in a market-driven organization, on the basis of their business development and customer satisfaction performance.

This represents the next stage of evolution for healthcare managers. In the past, their purview was expanded from simply clinical management to include financial management responsibilities. Head nurses in hospitals, for example, are not only responsible for the clinical performance of their staff, they are also responsible for the development and managing of budgets and the use of resources. As an organization more clearly appreciates the volume part of the business equation (volume times price = revenue less costs = profit) a commensurate emphasis is placed on business development as is placed on financial control issues. Then line managers are given an expanded set of responsibilities: clinical, financial, and marketing responsibilities. The one who can grow a particular line of business is the manager at the helm of that line of business. (See Chapter 6 on Service Line Management, Marketing, and Managed Care.)

- Just as a management team becomes more sophisticated in handling its financial management responsibilities, to the degree that it has excellent leadership from a chief financial officer, so also a management team becomes more sophisticated in handling its marketing management responsibilities if it has an effective leader in the role of the chief marketing officer. Over time, a healthcare organization sees its managers come to understand their fixed and variable costs. A well-managed organization financially is able to use flexible budgets—if a department is developing more profit than expected in a given time period, it receives more resources so that it can continue an upward path. So also, a **more sophisticated management group** begins to know how to pinpoint the lush, underserved segments in its marketplace and to make the quick adjustments and improvements that take advantage of those underserved segments.

- Just as financial information systems are developed to provide managers across an organization with the timely information they need to effectively handle their financial management responsibilities, so also the marketing executive makes sure that managers have **timely marketing information**. Information concerning how business is coming in the door and which segments are producing the most volume and return becomes golden information for managers. Organizations, for example, that never tracked referring physician information now make sure that they know precisely where every referral is coming from, and watch and try to influence referral trends. Managed-care companies become very adept at knowing exactly which companies are providing them with the largest book of business and what steps make a difference in influencing employer and employee groups. There is a tight feedback loop from strategy to impact to results and back to revised strategy.

- Just as there is a quarterly review of progress towards financial objectives at the board level, in a powerful marketing-oriented organization there also will be a **quarterly review of progress towards business development objectives** at the board level.

The healthcare marketing executive makes many other contributions to the success of the organization than just this set of culture transforming initiatives. Marketers play many roles in their own right. In this, too, marketing is similar to finance.

Just as the finance function provides specialized services to the organization that are outside and in addition to its investment in the financial management system of the organization—such as managing arbitrage, performing financial modeling, securing favorable access to capital, etc.—so also the marketing function provides specialized services that go beyond the marketing management system—such as managing media relations, conducting ad campaigns and marketing research, producing print communications, etc.

Healthcare executives reflecting on the way finance has been woven into the texture of healthcare organizations' culture not only have reason to take heart, they can see a roadmap of what they need to emphasize and accomplish. Not only can an initially foreign management discipline be introduced and inserted into the healthcare's organization culture, it can eventually become one of its driving values. If finance can do it, so can marketing.

Healthcare marketing executives will be effective, if—with the blessing and support of the CEO—they reach for and use the power of the organization's calendar, clear a space for marketing, and make it the subject of an entire management system.

Strategy #3: Provide opportunities for operating units across the organization to learn marketing through doing marketing

Exposing line managers and physicians across a healthcare organization to the management discipline of marketing carries with it its own power to persuade and incentive to change, because the practice of marketing, by its very nature, is discovery-filled and practically profitable. The experience of authentic marketing, therefore, catches professionals up and changes them. The challenge, therefore, to the healthcare executive is to find ways to introduce and involve colleagues in the practice of marketing. The best way to involve them is in areas of their own self-interest through the development of marketing plans for their programs and services.

The healthcare marketing executive, therefore, proceeds with marketing plans in a similar way that he or she proceeds with involving colleagues in the design, study, and use of market research: through demonstration, codification, and institutionalization. The healthcare executive first demonstrates what good marketing plans are and what they are not. He or she selects some high-profile examples and models effective marketing plans by taking control of the process and format for producing the plans in a way that is enjoyable for the participants, produces results in the market, and stimulates positive word-of-mouth within the organization. Secondly, the healthcare marketing executive, with the support of the CEO and the rest of the executive team, codifies marketing planning by making it an expected discipline for all key situations that require a significant investment of marketing resources. Finally, when an organization has reached full marketing maturity, the healthcare executive "institutionalizes" marketing plans, weaving them into the fabric of the way the organization is managed.

Demonstrate

The first step, then, in this strategy, is for the marketing function to demonstrate the power of "real" marketing planning and strategy development.

At the most elementary stages of developing this capability within the organization, the marketing staff plays a leadership role whenever particular requests come from the organization to the marketing department for promotion assistance.

The most simple example is the request for a brochure. It takes great delicacy and skill at this early stage of marketing's development for marketing staff members to successfully provide consulting services to line managers and physicians in this situation, because those line managers and physicians typically don't realize that they need consulting services. All they are asking for is a brochure. In their minds, this is a simple, straightforward request that should be complied with quickly and without fanfare or mugwumping. The marketing professional knows, however, that in order for a brochure to be effective, it needs to develop out of and be the result of a marketing-strategy thinking process.

The marketing staff person, therefore, has to be adept in laying out why certain questions have to be asked and answered in order for a brochure to be developed and produced. Namely:

- For whom is the brochure designed?

- What is the key benefit or benefits that that target market segment is looking for from the service?

- In what settings will the brochure be distributed?

Those three simple questions can make all the difference between a successful collateral piece and one that is a waste of money. By demonstrating to the requesting party how important each of those questions is through examples and implications coming out of the answers to the questions, the staff person can demonstrate the marketing behind the promotion.

A simple example: an obstetrics brochure—is it designed for the patient or for referring professionals? The tone, the content, and the level of investment will all hinge on the answer to that question.

What is the key benefit or benefits the target market segment is looking for from this service? A recent example: the obstetrics brochure designed for Misericordia Hospital in Philadelphia, demonstrates clearly the importance of asking this question on the front end. The draft content of the brochure as it was developed originally by clinical staff members didn't give priority to the issues the market was looking for. Instead, it presented the issues that occurred to the staff as top-of-mind and important. In thinking through the issues and needs of their target market, a number of benefits rose to the top and began to shape the content of the brochure. Issues concerning the level of training of the physicians, the attitude of the nurses, the attention to safety and security issues for the newborn, and the availability of pain management techniques were the four top issues identified by staff as concerns that they hear consistently from their customers. That whole "user train of thought" then shaped the content of the brochure. (See Exhibit 3-1)

Exhibit 3-1: Misericordia Hospital's "Blessed Beginnings"

Let Us Welcome Your Baby Into The World

A professional staff with a personal touch

Blessed Beginnings offers the services of Misericordia's skilled staff. Their primary concern is the health and comfort of mothers, their babies and families.

Physicians

Misericordia's board-certified obstetricians and gynecologists, pediatricians and specialists are uniquely qualified to provide quality care with compassion.

Nurse-Midwives

Misericordia's experienced nurse-midwives are certified in pregnancy and childbirth care. They are committed to making every woman's pregnancy a healthy first step toward parenthood.

Nursing Staff

Skilled professionals highly trained in newborn and maternal care provide continuity of care throughout each woman's entire birth experience.

The comfort of modern facilities

Single-Room Maternity Care

Labor, birth and recovery all occur in one room specially equipped with the most advanced equipment available.

LDRP (labor, delivery, recovery, post-partum) rooms were designed to offer the safest, most modern childbirth experience in a pleasant, comfortable environment.

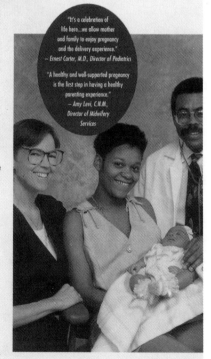

"It's a celebration of life here...we allow mother and family to enjoy pregnancy and the delivery experience."
– Ernest Carter, M.D., Director of Pediatrics

"A healthy and well-supported pregnancy is the first step in having a healthy parenting experience."
– Amy Levi, C.N.M., Director of Midwifery Services

Misericordia nurse educators provide assistance and support to family members.

Exhibit 3-1: Misericordia Hospital's "Blessed Beginnings" (continued)

The Support You Need From The Beginning

COMMUNITY

DIGNITY

EXCELLENCE

STEWARDSHIP

"We have implemented a program designed around community need, allowing us to develop ties with women before, during and after their pregnancies."
— Clinton Turner, M.D., Director of Women's Services

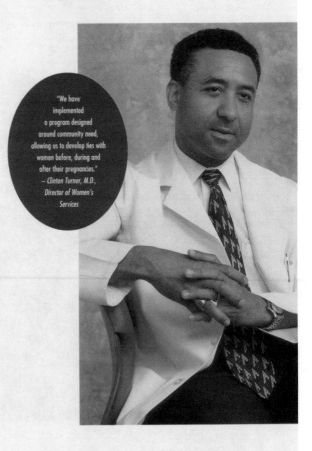

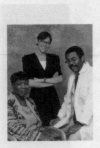

LDRP Nurse Manager/Nurse Educator Priscilla Murphy, Certified Nurse-Midwife Amy Levi and Dr. Ernest Carter are all committed to serving the needs of West Philadelphia's families.

Exhibit 3-1: Misericordia Hospital's "Blessed Beginnings" (continued)

Personalized prenatal care

Our staff is available to help women from the day they know they are pregnant. We provide routine physical examinations and lab tests, nutritional guidance, prenatal classes and personalized counseling. Women who are not pregnant can also access the guidance they need, to help ensure healthy future pregnancies through routine gynecological care.

Misericordia's nursing staff provide family-centered, family-focused care.

Our dedicated caregivers are unmatched in providing individualized health care that is family focused and community oriented. Women and their families will benefit from the care of the Blessed Beginnings Program before, during and after birth.

Family support

Specially trained nurse educators are available to assist fathers, too. All family members receive education about the woman's pregnancy and progress of the baby, as well as instruction on newborn and infant care.

Childbirth preparation

A skilled team of physicians, nurse-midwives, nurses, social workers, educators and nutritionists provide complete pregnancy and childbirth services. These experienced professionals are available to help support women and their families through the adjustments of being a new parent.

Family life programs

Misericordia's family programs offer classes throughout the year for the childbearing family. These include: Childbirth Education, Preparing For Birth, Motherwell® Maternity Fitness classes, Sibling classes, Expectant Grandparent classes and Baby Care Preparation.

Our staff: The Misericordia difference

Our physicians, nurse-midwives, nurses, social workers, counselors and educators are available to help at every stage of pregnancy and through labor. They are guided by their professionalism and respect for the dignity of the individual.

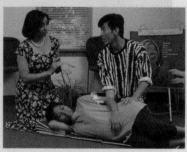

Misericordia's certified instructors offer training in childbirth preparation techniques.

Exhibit 3-1: Misericordia Hospital's "Blessed Beginnings" (continued)

Our Focus Is You And Your Baby

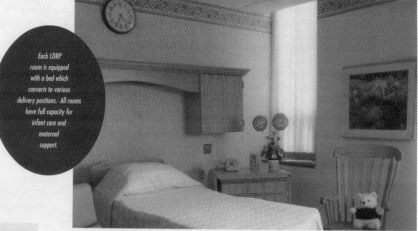

Each LDRP room is equipped with a bed which converts to various delivery positions. All rooms have full capacity for infant care and maternal support.

Additional services available through Misericordia

- Anesthesiology
- Antenatal testing unit
- Cesarean delivery
- Comprehensive nursery suite
- Laboratory studies
- Neonatal services including Level III NICU
- Ultrasound

A room of your own

We want women to feel as comfortable as possible through labor, delivery, recovery and post-partum. Each of our LDRP rooms is fully equipped to help provide the most personalized care in the safest, most pleasant surroundings. Mothers and babies will enjoy the comfort of these modern, attractive rooms until the end of their stay.

Family participation

Women will feel more relaxed when supported by their partners or family members during labor. We encourage partners and other support persons to participate during this special time in a woman's life.

Jacuzzi

We invite women to experience the relaxation of our Jacuzzi during labor. The pulsation of water against tense muscles enhances comfort and reduces pain for women in labor.

Breastfeeding Instruction

The services of skilled lactation consultants are available for women who choose to breastfeed their babies.

A state-of-the-art security system provides protection for all mothers and babies, and monitors all visits to the unit.

Finally, how will it be used and in what settings will it be distributed? The answer to this question determines the production values required of the piece and the quantity to be produced, which in turn determines the budget. Not to make these decisions is to render impossible the production of a brochure that is tightly targeted, convincingly written, and efficiently used. This simple example of an interactive process between clinical people and a marketing function can either be very enlightening or, if handled in an overly apologetic or overly officious way, can be destructive for the future development of a marketing consciousness. It is, however, typically a first step on the road.

These ad hoc encounters between marketing staff members and clinical management types either begin to spread a positive reputation for marketing or they begin to cast a gloom over the organization. If these moments of assistance around ad hoc projects turn out to be a satisfying experience for the line managers and physicians—one that is illuminating for them and not confusing—it will serve marketing well. This is no little achievement for marketing staff members. Most often, clinical people think they know what they want. They assume that the development of a brochure is a straightforward task. For the marketing professionals to attempt to open their minds to a bigger picture can be fraught with negativity. On the other hand, it is an important first step for marketing to take a clear stance vis-à-vis the discipline of developing effective marketing communications—while at the same time being supportive and responsive. It is the first step towards making marketing staff members not just order-takers, but recognized internal consultants and professionals.

Codify

A more important step, however, in this first stage of demonstrating the value and power of good marketing planning comes when the marketing executive is able to take the lead in the development of some key marketing plans for the organization.

This step assumes that the healthcare marketing executive has convinced senior management to call out a few priority marketing objectives for the organization and not make all requests for marketing services coming from all quarters of the organization equivalently important. This is an important turning point for marketing in a healthcare organization. Oftentimes, decisions concerning resources to be provided by the marketing function are determined through the squeakiest-wheel method. Those with the most political power in the organization or those who can make the most noise are the ones who receive resources and support from the marketing function.

The turning point is reached when the senior management team determines the four or five priority marketing objectives for the organization, in effect, signaling to the organization that first priority and first claim on resources will be given to these four or five priorities. This list of priority marketing objectives for the organization can be called the "marketing slate." They are "carved in stone." Once selected with care and deliberation, they are not easily changed. It is expected that they will remain the priorities—at least for a given year—knowing how challenging a task internally it will be to orchestrate their full achievement.

This marketing slate funnels resources where they will have the most effect on the marketplace, channels the marketing department's energies into the most productive areas of return, and protects the marketing staff members from the feeding frenzy from the multiple stakeholders within the healthcare organization for marketing time and resources. When the organization understands the organization's four or five priority marketing objectives—if marketing staff members are not able to respond to every request, it is not because they are unwilling or not hardworking. It is typically because they are fully engaged in supporting the four or five priorities of the organization.

It is at this point that the healthcare marketing executive can demonstrate clearly to the organization how to do marketing in an effective, head-turning, positive word-of-mouth fashion.

Institutionalize

The third step in having the organization learn marketing by doing marketing comes when the vice-president of marketing convinces the rest of his or her colleagues in administration to make the development of a marketing plan an annual expectation for all departments as they develop their annual departmental or service line plan.

Every department has customers. Most departments have internal customers. To identify the priority needs of their most important customers and develop a plan to improve their customers' satisfaction is indeed a marketing planning process. Using a simplified version of the

STRAP method, the whole organization begins to function in a marketing mode. (See Chapter 5, "Healthcare Marketing Plans That Secure Results: A Proven Method.")

A director of maintenance, for example, produced a marketing plan for his department. In it, he identified the nursing staff as a key customer and identified their frustrations with slow response to "minor repair issues" as being a stumbling block and a source of sour relations between maintenance and nursing. His response to the problem was not to reiterate "fill out a requisition." His response was to develop a "DIN" cart, a "Do It Now" cart that was pushed around the whole hospital every morning by "Danny the DIN man" who fixed whatever could be fixed in less than 20 minutes on the spot. In doing so, the director of maintenance eliminated the system of requisition. By deploying his resources more creatively, he was able to solve the problem. Instead of making "minor repairs" an end of the queue issue, he devoted one staff person to taking care of those issues in a focused amount of time.By attending to those "minor issues" quickly, he avoided more time-consuming, more expensive repairs later. Needless to say, he dramatically improved the reputation of maintenance with the nursing department.

The practice of the management discipline of marketing is appropriate for each and every department in a healthcare organization.

Strategy #4: Fight and win a few key battles over operations issues in the name of the customer

The fourth strategy for a healthcare marketing executive who desires to turn an organization in a fundamental way towards the customer is to use the existing structures of power in a focused way on behalf of the customer.

Frequently in a marketing plan, line managers and physicians begin to get somewhat leery about the issues coming to the fore through market analysis and research. The "product and place" issues are another way to say operational or clinical issues in the traditional management structure of health care. They may begin to ask, "What does this have to do with marketing?" They are, of course, equating marketing with promotion. It is at this moment that the healthcare marketing executive needs to be very adroit with political power. When issues emerge that are both critical for the marketplace in terms of satisfaction—and the traditional bailiwick of operations vice-presidents and physicians—the organization needs to make a choice. It can either decide to leave things as they are or to change because it recognizes the importance of the change in the eyes of the marketplace. The healthcare marketing executive is the person to force the issue and facilitate the change. He or she cannot make the change himself or herself. He or she depends on a close working relationship with the rest of the senior management team, the hierarchy of the medical staff, and most importantly, the chief executive officer.

Take, for example, the extended example used on pages 91–92 concerning standards of care for breast cancer. At one major hospital in the midwest, a leading surgeon worked for almost 10 years to have protocols developed that the surgery department would follow that were customer sensitive and friendly. He finally succeeded in having them accepted by the Department of Surgery—once the administration recognized their importance in terms of market development, and lent its backing to the struggle within the clinical department.

At another hospital, the Radiology Department resisted making changes that would make the mammography service much more customer-responsive and friendly. It took the threat of changing the hospital system's relationship and contract with the radiology group before the change was made. Better hours, board-certified radiologists explicitly trained in reading mammographies, faster reporting of results to physicians and women—these don't seem like earth-shaking changes. They were, however, not the way the radiologists were accustomed to working. The changes would disturb their vacation and time off schedules. They resisted making the changes until they received an ultimatum from administration.

Such high-level struggles say to the organization in a very clear way either, "We are intent on serving and satisfying customers," or, "We are intent on satisfying and serving ourselves." If it goes in favor of the customer, the organization deepens its commitment to the principles of marketing.

In another situation, a marketing executive, presenting the recommendations of a market research and planning consultation designed to upgrade the profile of the healthcare organization's services for women, was interrupted by a leading obstetrician who paid her a compliment. "I thought you were going to superimpose on us models of women's health programs that have worked elsewhere in the country. Instead, I can see that everything you are recommending comes right out of the research." The rest of the management team was shocked. This physician rarely gave compliments. The presentation resumed. A minute later, the marketer was recommending, "Reduce the C-section rate from 26 percent to below or at the national average." The same physician interrupted again, not with a compliment but this time with a sharp rebuke, "Wait a minute. What does that recommendation have to do with marketing? That's a clinical issue." The marketing person responded, "But Doctor, we just saw how important this issue is for managed-care companies, and we agreed how important managed care is for our future. Furthermore, women are increasingly asking about the C-section rate and making it one of their key issues when choosing an obstetric service."

Is the C-section rate only a clinical matter in this situation? Not for an organization listening to the voice of the customer. A healthcare executive who brings the voice of the market to the decision table is invaluable to the success of an organization. He or she will gain the respect of and a greater hearing for the customer and marketing as a management discipline, if he or she presses the customer's point of view in situations that demand change. If at times she/he is successful in facilitating such changes in the way the organization conducts business, she/he will rise very high in the organization's estimation.

CHAPTER 4

Upgrading a Hospital's Image: A Guide to Healthcare Positioning

INTRODUCTION

Many doors open to a hospital that has a strong, positive reputation in the community.

- Physicians find it easier to attract patients if they practice at a hospital that is preferred by the community. In turn, to the degree that a community prefers a hospital, to that degree it is easier to attract physicians to practice at that hospital.

- Specific clinical services such as cardiology, oncology, obstetrics, etc., are easier to grow if they are offered by a hospital that is already highly regarded by the community.

- Managed-care companies want to offer as part of their packages the hospital that is most highly valued by employers and employees in the community.

- Employees are heavily influenced in their choice of insurance packages by hospital reputation.

In all these ways, success in the marketplace begins and ends with a positive reputation or image.

A positive image can be made more positive. A negative image can be turned around. A low-watt identity can be dialed up. A best-kept secret identity can be revealed.

This chapter is for all those who seek a clearer, more positive image in the marketplace for their hospitals.

As we have seen in Chapters 1 and 2, a stronger reputation for a mainframe hospital contributes to securing additional managed care as well as fee-for-service business. It is an important focus of leadership attention in the old and new paradigms and in the era between the times.

This chapter also presents a step-by-step guide to the strategic marketing issue of positioning as it applies to healthcare. The in-depth example utilized is that of a hospital, but the methodology applies to other healthcare organizations as well.

The first order of business for an organization aspiring to strengthen its standing in the marketplace is to craft a positioning strategy for the organization; and make sure there is a name, themeline, and look that expresses the positioning strategy and an agreed-upon plan of action to emblazon the chosen positioning into the mind of the marketplace.

The positioning strategy is the first order of business for marketing because the organization's identity or image is its most important possession. Before the marketplace can choose a given hospital, it has to be positively disposed to that organization. A positive, believable image is fundamental for successful marketing. Positive name equity is as important for a hospital's survival as financial equity.

HOW A POSITIVE IMAGE CONTRIBUTES TO THE FINANCIAL WELL-BEING OF A HOSPITAL

1) A positive, believable image helps customers choose one hospital instead of another—to the degree that they have a say in the choice.

Increasingly, physicians indicate that when they are on more than one medical staff, they leave the choice of the hospital to the patient. Moreover, consumers indicate that for many services and in many situations, they indicate to the physician where they want to go. Finally, in many situations the consumer chooses the hospital first and looks for a physician on the medical staff of that hospital on a national level, it breaks down in the following ranges:

Question: What best expresses where and how you happened to be hospitalized?

40–50%	"My physician told me where to go."
30–40%	"My physician gave me options and we decided together." or "My physician gave me options and left it up to me."
10–25%	"I chose the hospital first and then the physician, based on hospital affiliation."
2–30%	"My insurance told me where to go."

While it is true that physicians hospitalize patients, it is important before concentrating all marketing attention and resources on physicians, to understand how decisions are actually made. The general public, employers, managed-care organizations, and physicians are all important constituents for the hospital's marketing program.

2) A positive, believable image makes it easier for physicians to recommend a particular hospital. If patients are positively disposed to a particular hospital, the physician is not embarrassed or loath to recommend that hospital. The more positively patients perceive the hospital, the more positively they regard the physician who is sending them there. That is why physicians frequently implore a particular hospital to upgrade its image and communicate more aggressively to the public.

In fact, at times, a negative hospital image is a heavy burden on individual staff physicians. A physician recounted how "patients would call my office and ask the receptionist what hospitals I served on. When she responded "X" hospital is the only hospital where Dr. practices, the inquiring potential patients frequently would hang up. End of discussion. The negative reputation of the hospital definitely hurts my practice."

3) A positive, believable image in the mind of the marketplace as a whole makes it much easier for a hospital to attract physicians to its staff. "My status as a physician is enhanced because of my staff privileges at this hospital. The reputation of the hospital and the

specialists on staff here reflects back on me. That's why I came to this hospital rather than to others."

4) A positive, believable image makes it easier for the marketplace to hear and accept claims and messages about particular services or new programs from the hospital. "It's hard for me to believe that that hospital can have an excellent heart program. We've heard negative things about it for years. We are much more likely to believe that the hospital in the next community has an excellent heart program because its overall reputation is so positive."

5) A positive, believable image enables a hospital to harness the power of the word-of-mouth networks in its area. One hospital, for example, that enjoyed a fine reputation in its service area was able to run the following ad: "When you want to know where the best hospital is, ask the experts . . . your neighbors." The hospital knew that word-of-mouth networks for newcomers meant that people would jump over other hospitals closer to their homes and come to their hospital because of the power of its reputation.

6) A positive, believable image supports successful fundraising efforts and is a hospital's best first line of defense against loss of not-for-profit status.

A hospital's reputation is as important as a lawyer's reputation, a priest's reputation, a restaurant's reputation, a therapist's reputation, or a child care center's reputation. If it is negative, the market will go out of its way to avoid you. If it is neutral, the market will find it difficult to notice you. If it is positive, the market will flock to you.

7) A positive reputation helps a hospital when managed-care companies are selecting institutions for their panels. It is hard for managed-care companies to leave out a well-regarded, preferred provider. It makes it harder for them to sell their products if they don't offer the market's preferred healthcare providers.

8) A positive reputation with those who are employed in the marketplace puts pressure on employers to make sure that they offer benefit package options that include employees' favored healthcare providers—to the degree employers want their benefit package to please and motivate their employees.

9) A positive hospital reputation has positive halo power for the managed-care option of which it is a part. Employees make the hospital reputation one of their key selection variables when they are choosing among benefit package options.

Given the importance of a hospital's image and reputation, is it possible to change a negative image to a positive one? Is it possible to change a neutral or bland image into a vibrant, positive one? Can a hospital's image and reputation be enhanced? The answer is "no," if the hospital's, its physicians', and clinical staffs' performances are indeed inferior. The answer is "yes," if the hospital's performance is better than its reputation.

How does one change or enhance one's image or reputation? The answer is through a marketing management discipline called *positioning*. Image is what you have. Positioning is what you choose.

POSITIONING: THE CONCEPT

Effective positioning strategy answers the questions: How do we want the marketplace to see us? How do we want to be perceived? As such, it is the public face of the mission statement. The mission statement states what an organization wants to *be*. A positioning statement articulates how an organization wants to be *perceived*. As such, it recognizes the critical importance of perception. In situations where those inside an organization bemoan the fact that they are perceived negatively—sure that their performance is indeed better than the marketplace perceives it to be—it is important for them to stop regretting the fact and to recognize that in many ways perception is all. The challenge is to bring consonance between reality and perception. Otherwise, the marketplace will not choose an organization over competitors.

A good positioning places the organization before the marketplace so that customers are seeing the institution in an illuminating, positive light. This angle of perception creates and reinforces a perception of the organization that gradually assures current and potential customers that it is the place for them.

A Positioning Strategy Must Fulfill Three Requirements to Be Effective

1) It must differentiate the organization from competitors.

A "me too" positioning will only benefit the people who said it first. The public will assume it's coming from them. If the niche that is staked out in the mind of the marketplace is already occupied by others, the organization will continue to be lost in the clutter.

2) The positioning has to reflect a quality or attribute that is valued by the marketplace.

If the positioning doesn't reflect an important value to the marketplace, it will not provide enough reason for the marketplace to choose you instead of others. It won't prompt behavior change or change minds.

3) The positioning has to be based on a fundamental strength or strengths of the organization.

You can't fool the public through puffery. If the reach of the positioning outstrips perceived performance, the organization holds itself up to potential ridicule. When United Airlines, for example, changed its look, colors, and logo to express its new status as a global carrier, it reflected a change that was real and recognized by the marketplace. It enhanced its positioning. On the other hand, when Ford began to hold up its rather clunky Escort car as "a world-class automobile," it held itself up to some derision. Even more, the hospital that began describing itself as a "world-class hospital," produced disbelieving shakes of the head in the marketplace. Or the small community hospital that saw an opening in the market and began describing itself as the "Medical Center of X County" produced a derisive "What, them?" reaction from the marketplace.

Before Developing an Effective Positioning Strategy, Pause and Reflect on the Difficulties of Changing a Hospital's Image

There are three important facts about the marketplace that make it difficult to effectively reposition a hospital.

1) A hospital's reputation is rooted in real-life stories people tell about the hospital every day.

Very few institutions in society are discussed the way hospitals are discussed. What happens in the parking lot, in the emergency room, when somebody receives the bill, when they visited, when they lay in a bed—what happened to them at those moments, and what they say to others, crystallizes into the hospital's image and reputation. If what happens in those moments is positive, the hospital has a positive reputation. If what happens in those moments is negative, the hospital has a negative reputation.

Think, for example, of the marketing consultant who, after getting off a plane in Daytona Beach, Fla., heard his taxi driver (frequently an important source of market information and a reliable source of impressions) say, "When I first came to Daytona Beach, there was nothing but the high school and the hospital."

The consultant saw the opportunity for some informal market research. He asked "Is the hospital a large hospital?"

The taxi driver said, "Oh, we've got a number of hospitals now."

"Which one is the best?"

He answered, "There's a lot of fighting about that in this community. A lot of disagreement."

"Which one do *you* think is best?"

"X Medical Center," he answered.

"Why?" the consultant asked, hoping that he would hear some insights into how an ordinary person on the street makes such a global judgment from afar.

He answered, "The high-tech equipment. You wouldn't believe their laboratories. But I understand, when you're going to have a baby, you don't want to go there because they mix them up."

Now, where did that story start? How did this taxi driver hear that the hospital had mixed up some babies? How did this come to influence his attitude towards the hospital? From word-of-mouth stories that create the hospital's reputation.

The same consultant received a call from a neighbor that his daughter Molly had fallen off her bike and gashed her chin. He went running down the block to where she was and saw immediately that she did, indeed, need stitches to close the gash. He said, "Molly, we're only a few blocks from the closest emergency room. Let's get over there."

Molly froze and said, "No way. I don't want to go to that emergency room. I've heard too many bad things about that emergency room." She was nine years old at the time.

He said, "Molly, we'll have to call to get your mom to come over with the car and go all the way across town to the other hospital's emergency room."

She said, "I don't care, that's what I want to do."

Of course, that is what they did. A nine-year-old has a strong impression of a particular hospital because of the word-of-mouth stories that she has heard.

The only way, therefore, that one can effectively turn around a reputation in a fundamental way is to change those word-of-mouth stories.

When a young CEO took over a community hospital in Wisconsin, one of his first moves was to complete a market research study to get a handle on why there had been slippage over the years. Focus groups conducted with former users of the emergency room indicated very clearly to him that the emergency department experience was producing a negative set of stories about the hospital in the marketplace. He braved the political fallout from firing an entrenched group of emergency room physicians and brought in a new set of board-certified emergency room physicians. That was his first step in successfully changing the image and reputation of the hospital. He had little chance of altering the hospital's reputation as long as he allowed the sources of negative word-of-mouth to stay in place.

2) People know what they know.

Once a particular image or reputation has been established, it is very difficult to unseat. The only way to change the reputation is to fill the channels of communication with new information and new stories.

When another young CEO came to an Illinois hospital, he also heard negative stories about his emergency room through consumer research, but with a difference from the Wisconsin hospital example. These comments reflected old horror stories, not fresh ones. The stories were being repeated even after the hospital had actually improved its performance. The hospital hadn't dislodged the old stories with up-to-date ones.

In this case, the answer was not to replace the emergency physicians but to fill the channels of communication with new messages. He and his staff placed a series of ads and stories about recent developments in the emergency room—how waiting times had been reduced, the board certification credentials of the emergency room physicians, how the staff had handled the victims of a major train accident, etc. As a result, the quality rating of the hospital in the next community attitude survey jumped dramatically within a year—especially among residents who had lived in town for over five years. It was not changing performance that was the response to a negative reputation in this case, but filling the channels of communication with more up-to-date messages.

3) Our culture has a well-developed ability not to notice.

So many messages wash over us every day that we develop an uncanny ability to not let them get through to us. If we let all the messages sent our way every day connect in our brains, we most likely would short circuit.

Consequently, any advertiser trying to reach us or reposition its product in our minds is actually competing with all the others in the communications channels hawking their wares. Only the very best break through to us. Either they touch some intensely felt need, or by sheer creativity, catch our attention and slip past our defenses.

Consequently, any hospital trying to reposition itself in the mind of the marketplace is swimming through the same clutter as everyone else. It is competing for the attention of the marketplace with the best and most creative marketers in our culture. The competitors for share of mind in this case are not only other hospitals but also Nike, Apple, and McDonald's.

In order to be effective, our repositioning efforts have to be so disciplined and so well executed that we break through the competitive communication clutter.

Those involved in healthcare notice healthcare communications. That's because they are in the business and already attuned. The rest of the marketplace? They notice only by dint of sheer creativity, because we meet a felt need or through repetition, i.e., the "drip, drip method." It is most effective to do all three at once.

It is not easy to reposition a hospital in the mind of the market. Nonetheless, as we shall see, it can be done.

How to Recognize an Effectively Positioned Hospital

A hospital that has done an effective job of positioning itself has these characteristics:

1) Leadership has crafted a positioning statement.

2) A well-positioned hospital has a well-utilized themeline.

3) A well-positioned hospital has a name that expresses as accurately as possible the chosen positioning statement.

Leadership Has Crafted a Positioning Statement.

How a positioning statement differs from, but is not identical to, a mission statement.

In brief, the mission statement articulates what the organization wants to be, whereas the positioning statement articulates how the organization wants to be *perceived*.

The mission statement makes explicit the organization's values, roles, services, the preferred constituencies it serves, and the spirit in which it serves them. It is typically a document of about a page in length. At times, it runs to many pages.

The positioning statement on the other hand is much briefer, no longer than a few sentences. It presents the core elements that will be the market's "take" on the organization. Just as a person's identity precedes, is simpler than, and is the wellspring for the person's motives, accomplishments, and aspirations, so also is the identity of an organization. *Who* the organization is rather than *what* it is.

For example, a university hospital's positioning statement reads as follows:

> We want to be perceived as the place where a continued stream of important medical breakthroughs is taking place. Because of the quality of our research and faculty, because we are in touch with the latest, we are the place where anyone who is seriously ill should prefer to come.

This statement is much briefer than its mission statement, which states everything from its three-fold role of research, teaching, and patient care, to its commitment to regional continuing education and its commitment to serving the disadvantaged to its attitude towards employees and taxpayers.

A suburban hospital's positioning strategy reads as follows:

> We want to be perceived as the finest hospital in our growing, affluent county.

Its mission statement, on the other hand, went on for a full page.

What are the benefits of a positioning statement?

1) An effective positioning statement allows an organization to move in one direction instead of fragmented in multiple directions.

Developing a formal positioning statement frequently brings to the surface the unspoken and at times competing visions of the organization's identity that various members of leadership possess. Unspoken and buried, those competing visions often have the effect of stymieing the organization and freezing it in place. Beneath the political wrangles that afflict many organizations are, without anyone quite realizing it or giving it voice, competing visions of identity. By comparing the competing visions in the context of an objective appraisal of an organization's history, values, capabilities, competitive situation, and marketplace needs, those that don't fully match the facts are revealed with their pluses and minuses. As a result of the ensuing dialogue, agreement can be forged, horizons adjusted, and a common vision embraced—unfreezing the organization.

A common debate, for example, within hospital leadership teams, revolves around the "community hospital identity" prized by some and the "regional referral identity" prized by others. Developing a positioning statement raises all the underlying feelings and issues, and provides a forum for coming to an enriched consensus. The end result is different and better than the individual parties might have expected. The organization as a result is not pulled in competing directions any longer but can move in one direction—the one that makes the most strategic and organizational sense.

2) An effective positioning strategy answers the longing within an organization through all levels of staff for a clear statement of identity.

In many organizations, one frequently hears the statements "Who exactly are we?" "Are we trying to be all things to all people?" "What are we going to be when we grow up?" "What do we stand for?" Even in situations where leadership has developed a strategic plan and communicated it to the organization, one still hears these laments. Having a strategic plan and a mission statement evidently doesn't fill the gap and longing for a sense of identity.

If the positioning strategy is on target it will express the unspoken aspirations and underlying pride of the staff in the organization. Staff members feel, once the identity has been given voice, "Yes, that is, of course, who and what we are."

A copywriter who worked on an assignment for Venture stores—a value-priced retail chain in the Midwest—had developed a themeline to express Venture's position in the market, which was a slightly higher-priced niche than K-Mart with a higher class of goods and more customer service. The themeline was: "Save at Venture. Save with Style." He asked before launching the campaign if he could talk to a cross section of store employees. He realized in talking with them that no one had ever communicated to them what Venture's position in the market was. As a result, before launching the external campaign, Venture conducted an intensive, internal campaign. Employees began to lift their heads in pride and reinforced with customers what proved to be a very successful external campaign.

3) A well-crafted positioning strategy renders all subordinate business and market development decisions easier to make and orchestrate.

The positioning strategy helps guide subsequent competitive moves and purchase decisions, not just marketing communications. Among them are:

- MD recruitment;
- clinical service investments;
- master site planning;
- service line choices;
- equipment purchases; and
- community outreach.

All hinge on the fundamental question: How do we want to be perceived by the market? This provides a helpful litmus test of important decisions. Does this move reinforce, undercut, or have little relation to our positioning strategy in the marketplace?

For example, a teaching hospital that was positioning itself as a cooperative, regional referral center for smaller hospitals jumped on the opportunity to lead the development of a primary-care physician recruitment and resource center *on behalf of the region*. It deepened its positioning and made it more vivid.

Another hospital that decided it would *not* be an across-the-board tertiary center, found it easier to concentrate on a limited set of four centers of excellence, and for the first time in its history refused certain capital requests from physician specialists outside of those four areas.

A university hospital, already perceived as a leading research center, began to position itself as a customer responsive institution. It recruited and featured a four-star chef who was quite visible in his tall white chef's hat as he traveled the halls responding in person to individual patient requests or complaints. Faculty saw him as a contributing part of the repositioning strategy.

4) A clear positioning strategy is fundamental for effective and efficient marketing communications.

Marketing, especially marketing communications, depends on consistency and repetition. All marketing communications with a clear positioning strategy in place can be coordinated to hammer home, time after time, the chosen identity in the mind of the marketplace.

A consistent look, theme, and tone in all communications from print to broadcast, in and of itself, begins to bring the positioning home.

Witness the introduction, or "launch," of the Mark VIII Lincoln. All the print and broadcast reinforce the theme "Try everything else first" and convey Ford's no-apology, confident positioning of the car as superior to the Japanese and German autos in its price class.

Furthermore, every creative execution of a communications element receives an important first screen. The positioning strategy serves as the first diagnostic tool for evaluating creative work. Pull the positioning statement out of the drawer, read it, and then ask—"Does this creative reinforce, undercut, or have nothing to do with our positioning strategy?

For example, an ad agency brought in a series of ads for a Center for Breast Health campaign. The positioning strategy: The center wanted to be perceived as the place that understands the fears and desires of women, listens sensitively to those fears, and brings to bear the very best in clinical competences to treat breast disease.

The first ads printed by the agency came across in focus group tests as sexist and indelicate in the way they talked about women's breasts. The ads were not approved and the agency had to start over.

A Well-Positioned Hospital Has a Well-Utilized Themeline.

Whereas, the mission statement is published and hung on as many walls as possible, the positioning statement is not published. As leadership's statement of strategy to itself, it is not communicated to the marketplace in its narrative form. Instead it is first transmuted into a memorable, telegraphic, emotion laden themeline. That is the form in which it will be communicated to the marketplace.

For example, the themeline of the University of Michigan Hospitals, "Knowledge Heals" is used consistently in all communications from the University of Michigan Hospitals. The essence of the organization, what differentiates it in the marketplace, and what makes it a place for the marketplace to prefer is communicated in two brief, packed words.

A themeline is used for the following three reasons:

1) It forces an organization to go on record in a public way. In some ways it forces an organization to be honest. It can no longer be all things to all people if it has staked out a positioning in a public way.

2) It translates complex ideas into a simple form that has a chance to break through the clutter. For example, "When it rains, it pours" is Morton Salt's theme.

A well utilized themeline will serve as a constant accompaniment to other more complex messages, tying them back to a consistent identity. The marketplace will not notice a didactic statement about an organization. It may, however, notice and let register a frequently used, penetrating themeline.

3) A themeline communicates to the heart, the emotions, and the imagination as well as to the mind.

For example, Federal Express' positioning statement may read:

Federal Express wants to be perceived as the most dependable delivery service in the business making sure that messages and packages deemed important to clients are delivered in a guaranteed, trackable way within an agreed-upon time, usually the next day from most locations, at a fair price.

Handed over to the copywriters that positioning statement became "When it absolutely, positively, has to be there overnight"— touching the nerve of anyone who has ever felt an equivalent sense of urgency over a package or letter.

Another example—a Tennessee psychiatric hospital's positioning statement read something like:

We want to be perceived as the cluster of talents that best understands mental illness, what it does to individuals and their families, and that knows best how to restore those afflicted to productive lives—within the limits of their illness.

The themeline: "Gentle treatment for troubled lives," which touches the right chords.

A good themeline depends on a clear positioning statement and solid conceptual thinking. An incisive positioning statement is produced by good analytic and strategic thinkers—the CEO/ marketing executive types. But when it comes to communicating the positioning, the baton is passed to the creative talents, the copy writers, to work their alchemy on the narrative stew to come up with a golden shaft of an identity line that will reach the heart and emotions as well as the brain.

It is at that level that attitudes can be changed and behavior influenced.

A Well-Positioned Hospital Has a Name That Expresses as Accurately as Possible the Chosen Positioning Strategy.

Most often the organization's name is so well established and already has so much equity in the marketplace that nothing else needs to be said—don't touch the name.

Other times, some adjustments in the name are dictated by the positioning strategy. Each of the terms—for example, "general," "community," "regional," and "medical center"—stake out particular niches in the mind of the marketplace.

One well-regarded hospital, for example—which in the past three years had purchased and was operating a rehabilitation hospital on its main campus, a psychiatric hospital on a campus two blocks away, as well as two major physician office buildings on a contiguous site all with distinct names—recognized it was time to change its name to "medical center" and tie all of those previously disparate identities under one umbrella, lending the halo effect of its name to them while maintaining as appropriate distinct names for each part. Signs and systems were put in place to support the power of the enhanced entity and identity.

Often times, these days two or more institutions have come together and there is a need for a new name. The name can either be developed apart from strategic considerations or more appropriately, as a result and expression of the positioning strategy.

Selected Special Questions Relating to Names

1) Should there be a multiplicity of distinct names for multiple services?

Some feel that a multiplicity of distinct names for services confuses the marketplace and dilutes the identity of the sponsoring organization. Do all the heart, cancer, diabetes, gastro, women's, psych, orthopedics, etc., services need to be named as well?

Naming a service makes sense only at a certain stage of maturity. For example, providing a distinct name such as "X" Cancer Center indicates to the market that the service has evolved from just specialty doctors to care for patients and beds to care for them in. It also indicates that the organization along with its physicians has developed a multidisciplinary program on behalf of the patients that integrates the contributions of nurses, related ancillary services, and at times, other physician specialties that can include protocols for patient education, case management, prospective care planning, and staff development. A distinct name can mean the caregivers are not shifted from the care of one type of patient to another, but are dedicated to and fully trained in caring for the specific disease or condition. Finally, it can mean—and this makes the term "center" particularly appropriate—that the care is given in a dedicated place with distinct access and inquiry points such as patient care information and scheduling line.

In such a case, a distinct name is pointing to something important and real. A distinct name doesn't make sense and will be experienced as empty puffery if there is no program being named.

More to the point, giving a distinct name to a clinical service—if the service has matured as described—reflects a more adequate understanding of how healthcare decisions are made. A person with cancer or heart disease or an orthopedic problem is a distinct customer with distinct needs and decision variables. If a provider addresses those customers in terms of those distinct needs and decision variables, instead of generically, the provider stands a better chance of making a connection with those potential customers.

The hospital is the generic umbrella organization for a number of distinct services—in effect distinct businesses—because they have distinct customers with distinct decision-making variables. Specifically naming and featuring, for example, a cancer care service connects with those specifically looking for the best in cancer care. That potential patient wants to know if the organization is

A Case Study: Strategic Implications of a Naming Decision

What's in a name? A rose is a rose . . . Consider, for example, the advantages and disadvantages of Humana's decision—before it split its hospital and HMO lines of business, and before it merged into Columbia/HCA–to have all its hospitals across the country carry the same name, "Humana." The positives at first blush seem to outweigh the negatives and to make the decision seem a wise marketing move.

Advantages

The word "Humana," containing as it does the word "human," has a positive resonance for most people, communicates the positive side of the company's healthcare mission, and does not put front and center the corporate, for-profit side of the company's identity.

- With all the hospitals sharing the same name, the company takes a brand name approach, à la McDonald's. The marketplace should therefore expect:
  - a common level of quality, and a common style and set of policies and procedures no matter which Humana hospital across the country one enters; and
  - strong support from a central office with a national franchise and reputation to protect.
- Whenever something good or newsworthy happens to one part of the company or at one location, all the locations share in that development and story, e.g., Humana in Louisville and the news of the development of an artificial heart.
- The many locations with one name provide a national distribution network for a national managed-care product.

Disadvantages

- Whenever bad publicity affects one part of the company or one location, it affects to some degree all the others.
- It minimizes the local identity of each hospital and misses the way hospital decisions are usually made. People do go into McDonald's restaurants in many locations. Except in cases of emergency when traveling in multiple locations, the hospital purchase decision is made on a local basis. The more a given hospital in a given location is perceived as tied to, concerned about, and caring for a local community, the more successful the hospital will be in utilizing the word-of-mouth networks that are fundamental to healthcare marketing. This is especially true for the type of hospitals Humana owned, which are typically community as opposed to teaching or tertiary-care facilities.

If a hospital has few links or ties to a local community—not even through its name—it will have that much more difficulty gaining dominant market share, especially if it has competitors who *do* have those ties that bind.

In conclusion: every name is an expression of strategy. Either intentionally or unintentionally, a name stakes out some position in the mind of the marketplace.

particularly adept at and organized around the treatment of the cancer patient and doesn't care as much about the generic claims of the hospital as a whole. Of course, the overall reputation of the sponsoring organization helps potential patients believe the claims about its competency in cancer treatment, but it is for the latter that the potential patient is looking and around that that the purchase decision will be made.

Such an approach underscores the importance of the turn to service-line management hospitals have been taking and the importance of breaking the umbrella organization into its separate business units to better correspond to how the marketplace perceives, evaluates, and decides. It follows, therefore, that the stronger and more distinct each of the key services under the umbrella, the better. The more named services the hospital offers, the more customer segments with whom it has a chance of connecting. A designated Sports Medicine Center by that very name is closer to the customer than a hospital (that may or may not have orthopedic surgeons on staff, who may or may not have specific competencies in sports medicine, who the market may or may not think of to call for a reference, etc.). And the same holds true for other conditions or maladies.

The market is not confused by many different named services because in many ways there is really no such thing as a market in these situations. There are instead market segments. The segment looking for sports medicine help will notice and perhaps respond to the presence of a sports medicine center, but will probably not notice the message from the same hospital about the cancer center because that is not a need or a concern of that segment—and vice versa for the cancer patient.

Confusion can be minimized and a certain synergy achieved, however, if the identity of each named service or center is tied back to the sponsoring organization through look, signage, graphic standards, and repetition of the theme line.

Bishop Clarkson in Omaha, Nebraska, for example, concluded each message and each component of its four-year roll-out campaign with the phrase, "Once again, another first from Nebraska's first hospital." Distinct television commercials for

Clarkson's obstetrics, cancer, senior care, and heart services each ended with the theme, reinforcing the overall positioning of the sponsoring organization. Each of the featured services grew and Clarkson as a whole moved from fifth to second in that market-place over those four years.

2) Should the name of the hospital or the name of the service be given top billing?

It depends on which entity will give more leverage to the other. Putting the name of the hospital first connotes that the service is a function or department of the hospital rather than a service with some independent status of its own. At times, that is the accurate depiction and is the appropriate order.

Other times, especially in a situation where there are referrals to the service from other facilities, and especially if the hospital does not usually receive referrals for other clinical services from those referring facilities, it makes more sense to put the hospital in a second or subordinate position, e.g., "X" Heart Center at "X" hospital. That communicates that the facilities are referring to this service and doesn't imply an across-the-board commitment to that hospital for other clinical referrals.

3) Does the hospital name need to be specifically included in the name of the service?

Usually it is to the advantage of a given service for it to be linked by name to the sponsoring organization.

The hospital name communicates that the service is offered by a mainline medical organization, stable and trustworthy. It is not fly-by-night or sponsored by anyone unsavory.

The service, therefore, shares in the accreditation and societal standing of a mainframe hospital. If, for example, a hospital named its women's program, "The Women's Health Center," and not the Women's Health Center of "X" Hospital, the market would be forced to sort out such questions as—is this an alternative type health center or mainline medicine? Is it an abortion clinic? Who owns it and what are they after? Linking it to the hospital avoids those questions.

Linking a service by name to the hospital typically lends the credibility and name equity of the hospital to the service. One major university hospital in the Chicago area sponsored an employee contest to come up with a name for its new rehabilitation program. The winning entry was "Windy City Rehab." They were about to launch the program with that name and with no reference to the sponsoring organization, until wiser heads prevailed and the program was named more prosaically but much more effectively as "X" University Rehabilitation Center, using instead of ignoring all the credibility and power of this world-renowned institution.

There are some rare situations in which the hospital name could be left out of the name of the service:

- when the hospital's reputation is such that it will be better for the service if the service stands at arm's length;

- when the service is a service for which a hospital has little or no credibility, e.g., some wellness programs or cost containment programs for industry; and

- when a service is intended to actively involve specialists who are on staffs of hospitals that are traditional competitors of the sponsoring hospital.

POSITIONING: HOW TO DEVELOP AN EFFECTIVE POSITIONING STRATEGY

Steps to Avoid in the Development of a Positioning Strategy

The Meaning of the Terms "Leading" or "Best" Hospital Is Not the Same in All Markets.

In Boston and some other cities, for example, the terms "leading" or "best" hospital have a definite content and are ascribed to university teaching hospitals. In other markets—such as Cincinnati, Kansas City, and Minneapolis—"best" hospital status is not ascribed to the university hospital. In smaller cities, suburbs, and rural areas, "best" hospital status is ascribed to hospitals that don't even have teaching programs.

Just because a hospital is not a university or teaching hospital does not mean that, in its market, it can't pursue a #1 hospital strategy.

"Quality" Is Not a Univocal Term When Used to Describe a Hospital; It Is Definitely Not Just Another Way of Saying "Hi-Tech."

"Quality" is not a univocal term when ascribed to a hospital. It is multivariate. Moreover, it is definitely not synonymous or equated with hi-tech.

When the marketplace makes a judgment that a hospital is a quality hospital, it actually uses a number of indicators. Some of the indicators are more predictive in a mathematical sense than others and contribute more strongly to the marketplace's perceptions that a given hospital is a quality hospital. They are arranged in the following hierarchy:

1) The hospital is perceived to have quality physicians on its medical staff.

   This variable is by far the strongest correlative to the overall judgment of quality by the general public.

2) The hospital is perceived to offer "good care."

   Comprising this variable, which is almost as slippery as the term quality, are sub-meanings and judgments, i.e., the hospital staff is caring, attentive, adequately staffed, listening, and responsive.

3) The hospital is perceived to have quality nurses.

   Most people who have been hospitalized equate the quality of their hospital stay with the quality of the nursing care. They experience the nurses close-up and round the clock.

4) The hospital is perceived to care for highly specialized cases and to care for the very sick.

   The train of thought is that if a hospital can successfully care for the very ill, it surely can take care of the not so very ill.

5) The hospital is perceived as having the latest in high-technology equipment.

   Having heard the stories of technological breakthroughs, the tools of diagnostic wizardry, and the stories of people who were once deemed hopeless and who can now be healed, coupled with the tangibility of high-tech equipment—one either has it or not—makes this an important indicator of quality.

6) The hospital is perceived to have modern and up-to-date facilities.

A shining, new facility indicates to the public that investments are being made and commitments are being kept. Many hospitals that open new replacement facilities or new pavilions experience a spurt in business—almost from that very fact.

7) The hospital is perceived to be the place where the next generation is being taught.

Teaching programs communicate a number of things. The public understands that those who teach young professionals will be pushed to stay ahead and on their toes; that teaching something is a very fine way of making sure one understands it; and that those who teach are touched by a degree of altruism.

The public understands that those who teach are closer to the hearth of research and the latest discoveries than those who haven't cracked a professional book since they last took an exam. The time clinicians spend preparing to teach and in teaching is time away from making money. Those who teach are perceived, therefore, as motivated by values other than monetary. Presumably those other values make them more human, more willing to go the extra mile, and better caregivers.

On the other hand, teaching programs have a downside symbolism. If not managed, they can indicate that physicians in training—rather than full-fledged attendings—are the caregivers; that patients can expect interruptions from a range of anonymous healthcare workers; that patients will be guinea pigs for research and teaching; and that patients will be treated as numbers rather than persons.

8) The hospital is perceived as innovative and has a vigorous leader at the helm.

If the general public is constantly hearing about new developments at a particular hospital—given the underlying American faith in progress, e.g., if it's new, it's upward bound—the public begins to equate that with ever-improving. Moreover, recognizing the importance of leadership in any field, if hospital leadership is visible and capable, it is presumed that those qualities will eventually be embodied in the institutions that person leads. "Any great institution is, in its origin, the shadow of a great person."

9) The hospital is perceived as tuned in to the greater good and life of the community.

This perception reinforces a quality judgment, apparently by way of the principle of "noblesse oblige." In that spirit, the elite are expected to give back to society by the very fact that they have been given so much.

The principle is practiced, not just in Europe, but also in this country. For example, the American-elite Harrimans, Kennedys, DuPonts, and Rockefellers, in their second and third generations, dedicate themselves to public service. Their fortunes are established and it is time to give back to society. Analogously, if a hospital gives to the community in time, talent, donated leadership, and cooperative support to other agencies, it evidences a behavior that befits and is usually exhibited by those who have made their fortunes and who are among the elite. Through these behaviors the hospital is perceived to be an elite institution that is a "quality" place.

10) The hospital is perceived as supported by the movers and shakers in the community.

If the general public hears consistently that the chairs of boards of these major corporations—these well-known and wealthy community leaders—are involved on the board or committees or in fundraising efforts for a given hospital, a judgment is made. If those busy individuals judge the organization to be worth their time and talent, it must be a good place. Many organizations must be after them to serve on their boards and do fundraising. If they respond to that hospital, they must judge that it deserves their involvement more than other hospitals do. It must be a quality place.

Beware of Implications of the Multivariate Nature of the Term "Quality" as Ascribed to a Hospital.

A hospital can be perceived as high quality if it ranks high on some of the key variables, even if it doesn't rate highly on all of them. The way to be perceived as quality is to be perceived positively on those variables that contribute to the overall judgment of quality.

One can therefore "play" with one's reputation by playing with the perceptions of the subset variables. For example, strengthening one's board with heavyweight, high-profile community leaders can move the perception of quality up a notch or two but not have nearly the effect on the market's mind as the arrival on staff of a nationally renowned specialist. Developing a reputation for first-rate, satisfied, and caring nurses may influence the quality rating more effectively than being the first in the market to offer a new technology. Combining a number of moves designed to strengthen the perceptions on several criteria simultaneously will bring even more striking changes in a hospital's reputation and quality rating.

Hi-Tech/Hi-Touch Is Not the Only Continuum of Perception to Consider When Developing a Positioning Statement.

The marketplace looks at hospitals from many different angles. When asked, substantial parts of a market can make comparisons of hospitals using many points of comparison. Just as human beings perceive other human beings from multiple perspectives—depending on what's important to them—so also the marketplace snaps multiple shots of a hospital. To adequately understand how a hospital is perceived, what its profile in the market currently is, and to make decisions about the best way to reposition it, it makes sense to map how a hospital is perceived in comparison to competitors using all the coordinates the market uses. Taken together, those multiple shots shape the portrait of the hospital in the mind of the marketplace. That picture is the hospital's public "persona."

When forming their overall impression of a hospital, consumers come at a hospital vis-à-vis the issues that are most important to them, namely:

- quality,
- access,
- friendliness, and
- value or price.

To assess where a given hospital stands on these issues, one can ask the market to rate the hospitals in its area on each of the perception continua. Figures 4-1 through 4-4 illustrate sample ratings surveys for hospital quality, access, friendliness, and cost.

Moreover, the market observes each of these four issues from multiple angles. In Figure 4-1, for example, the issue of quality is appraised from at least the 10 different angles explained in the previous section.

Figure 4-1: Sample Ratings Survey for Hospital Quality

Quality	Highest	Lowest
Excellent medical staff	5 4 3 2 1	Poor quality medical staff
Good care	5 4 3 2 1	Poor care
Wonderful nursing staff	5 4 3 2 1	Poor nursing staff
Place to go when you're seriously ill	5 4 3 2 1	For "minor" illnesses
Latest, hi-tech equipment	5 4 3 2 1	Outdated equipment
New, attractive buildings	5 4 3 2 1	Old, outdated buildings
Full range of teaching programs	5 4 3 2 1	No teaching program
Innovative, progressive leadership	5 4 3 2 1	Old fashioned; behind the times
Involved with community	5 4 3 2 1	Removed from the community
Community leaders on the board	5 4 3 2 1	No involvement by community leaders

Figure 4-2: Sample Ratings Survey for Hospital Access

Accessibility	Highest	Lowest
Welcoming	5 4 3 2 1	Forbidding
Quick service	5 4 3 2 1	Long waits
Easy to find	5 4 3 2 1	Hard to find
Easy to use	5 4 3 2 1	Cumbersome paperwork/regulations
Easy to find one's way around	5 4 3 2 1	Difficult finding one's way

Figure 4-3: Sample Ratings Survey for Hospital Friendliness

Friendly	Highest	Lowest
Dedicated to serving others	5 4 3 2 1	Self-serving
Warm and friendly	5 4 3 2 1	Cold
Personal	5 4 3 2 1	Bureaucratic
Keep people informed	5 4 3 2 1	Never know what's going on
Responsive to patients	5 4 3 2 1	Staff's needs come first

Figure 4-4: Sample Ratings Survey for Hospital Cost

Cost	Highest	Lowest
Expensive	5 4 3 2 1	Low cost
Good value	5 4 3 2 1	Poor value

In addition to the four core issues of quality, accessibility, service, and cost, the market can and does compare hospitals by the specific services they provide—as in the hospital that does the best job providing heart services, obstetrics, etc. Those judgments also contribute to the hospital's overall "persona." To secure an accurate understanding of how hospitals are perceived and for what they are known, it makes sense to gather appraisals of hospitals by service. See Figure 4-5.

Figure 4-5: Sample Ratings Survey for Hospital Services

Center for Services	Highest	Lowest
Recognized cancer care center	5 4 3 2 1	No special identity in cancer care
Recognized heart care center	5 4 3 2 1	No special identity in heart care
Recognized diabetes care center	5 4 3 2 1	No special identity in diabetes care
Recognized emergency services center	5 4 3 2 1	No special identity in emergency services
Known for disease prevention and community education	5 4 3 2 1	Not known for disease prevention and community education
Recognized gastroenterology care center	5 4 3 2 1	No special identity in gastroenterology care
Recognized rehabilitation care center	5 4 3 2 1	No special identity in rehabilitation care
Recognized obstetrics care center	5 4 3 2 1	No special identity in obstetrics care
Recognized pediatrics care center	5 4 3 2 1	No special identity in pediatrics care
Recognized pulmonary care center	5 4 3 2 1	No special identity in pulmonary care
Recognized orthopedics care center	5 4 3 2 1	No special identity in orthopedics care

In many markets, an overwhelming percentage of the market has made judgments on all these matters, although they will have a clearer grasp on higher profile services. For lower profile services, however— such as mental health or ophthalmology—there are large percentages of "I don't know's," indicating that no organization in the market has yet captured the public's mind. The lack of mindshare can be as suggestive for positioning strategy as the presence of firmly established identities.

Finally, the market makes judgments not only about services hospitals provide but also by types of people served. They have impressions about the market segments the various hospitals care about and are organized to serve. See Figure 4-6.

Figure 4-6: Sample Ratings Survey for Hospital Target Patients

Target Patients	Highest	Lowest
Recognized for specially serving seniors	5 4 3 2 1	No special identity with seniors
Recognized for specially serving women	5 4 3 2 1	No special identity with women
Recognized for specially serving young, upwardly mobile adults	5 4 3 2 1	No special identity with young, upwardly mobile adults
Recognized for specially serving adolescents	5 4 3 2 1	No special identity with adolescents
Recognized for specially serving business	5 4 3 2 1	No special identity with business
Recognized for specially serving the poor	5 4 3 2 1	No special identity with the poor
Recognized for specially serving the working man/woman	5 4 3 2 1	No special identity with the working man/woman

When a hospital receives a particularly high or low mark in a particular area, it will most likely show up in the summation the marketplace makes about its character.

For example, one Catholic hospital ranked particularly low on the criterion "welcoming." The summary judgment of the hospital by the market was that it was cold, aloof, and rigid—very much contrary to the stated mission and values of the religious sisters that ran the hospital. Upon further investigation into how this reputation was being engendered in the general public, leadership realized that many of the first-impression moments were creating and reinforcing that identity. The very first encounter upon arrival was with an unsmiling security guard who insisted gruffly that each person coming in the door sign in, and the front entrance and waiting area were small, dowdy, and uncomfortable. Large signs giving curt directions seemed to be everywhere: "Only two visitors allowed at a time", "Each visitor needs a pass." And visiting hours were almost laughably short, especially in comparison to the visiting policies of the other hospitals in the area. In other words, a minor issue in an abstract sense—in comparison, for example, to the quality of physicians on staff—can become the hallmark of a current identity and a critical issue to address in the repositioning strategy.

All in all, there are at least 40 perception continua to use when attempting to get a fix on a given hospital's current image or persona in the marketplace. Hi-tech/hi-touch is definitely not the only one.

To limit the mapping of identity to simply the hi-tech/hi-touch polarity can be very misleading. It misses all the other angles from which the market perceives a hospital's identity, understates the range of competitive positioning options, and closes off promising lines of investigation for positioning strategy.

Moreover, the continuum "hi-tech/hi-touch" is inaccurate. Hi-tech is not the antipode to hi-touch. Hi-tech's antipode is low-tech. Hi-touch's antipode is distant, cold, aloof. Hi-tech and hi-touch are not opposite. They are two different continua of comparison and present two different traits.

In other words, to move towards hi-tech status is not to move away from hi-touch. Hi-tech/hi-touch in polarity implies that one can't do both at the same time. Because they are not opposites, but entirely distinct attributes, one can develop both at the same time.

Finally, the common phrase hi-tech/hi-touch reinforces the split in many providers' minds concerning quality health care, namely that there is some split possible between quality care and "good bedside manner," when the marketplace uses a broader definition of quality that insists on keeping them together. The marketplace insists that it isn't quality health care if it is not personal and responsive to the patient. There is no such thing as quality care that isn't hi-touch.

Some of the most successful examples of repositioning occur in situations where hi-tech/hi-touch are not understood to be in polarity.

The University of Missouri, for example, understood that the marketplace "gave" it the following attributes: serves the seriously ill, high technology, excellent medical staff. That is the *image* it had. To *position* itself more strongly—to strengthen its franchise and attract additional segments of business—it chose to position itself as the University hospital with a thorough culture of responsive, personalized customer service—beyond what any community hospital in the area provided. That is indeed now the way it is perceived by the marketplace—after years of from-the-ground-up work with staff and years of word-of-mouth stories from patients who were surprised and delighted by fine touches of personal service.

Phoebe Putney Memorial Hospital in Albany, Georgia, not long ago was known as the county hospital that serves the poor, in contrast to the private HCA hospital in town. Today, Phoebe Putney Memorial Hospital is repositioned as the hospital where most people in the market want to go for care and where many wish they could work. That repositioning occurred because leadership insisted that Phoebe Putney Memorial Hospital be known as the place with the latest in care and where exquisite, personalized care was delivered from first through final encounter.

Don't Try for Positioning That Is So Unique and Fresh That It Will Be New to Everyone in the Country.

Most effective positioning strategies make sense only in the context of the local competitive situation for which they are developed.

An executive with extensive experience in healthcare will probably have seen versions of a given positioning strategy elsewhere. There are only so many basic positioning strategies for a hospital. The challenge is not to develop a positioning that no one has ever seen before, as much as it is selecting a positioning that stakes out the niche in the mind of the marketplace that will provide the best competitive leverage. The audience for a positioning strategy is not other healthcare executives from other parts of the country, it is the leadership team in place in a given competitive situation.

For the leadership team in place, however, the positioning statement should be exciting because it will have an elegance of fit to the facts and a quiet power of promise. Leadership will sense that it strikes the chord in the market that will strengthen the franchise and generate additional business. That is not to say that the nuances of a given positioning statement might not be unique and the fine shadings fresh and intriguing. Moreover, the theme line will, if done well, have a fresh feel and immediacy of impact—even for someone outside the situation—because a themeline is a tool that cuts through the clutter with an element of emotional surprise and creative flair.

Take, for example, Shawnee Mission Medical Center (SMMC), in Johnson County, Kansas, just outside Kansas City. Johnson County has a well-insured and well-educated populace. In fact, it is the second wealthiest county in the whole country. Still growing, it has pride in its own independence. Instead of seeing itself as a mere bedroom community, it has a number of strong commercial and civic institutions that anchor and tie the community together. Its Junior College, for example, is rated the best in the country and has the regard and support of the whole community. Bill Cosby headlined a recent gala fundraiser.

SMMC is rated by citizens of the county as the finest hospital in the county. Over the past 10 years, it had steadily strengthened itself, and the community had noticed. Its emergency service, mental health, obstetrics, and wellness programs are rated the best in the area. Its heart program is seen as up and coming. It is rated best in terms of friendliness and nursing. For overall quality, it rates in their eyes second only to one other hospital in the whole Kansas City area—the big heart hospital in downtown Kansas City.

However, when its own management team members rated it in comparison to competitors in the region, they rated it lower than the community did. They had been so busy concentrating on improving the hospital that they barely realized what they had achieved.

Finally, three of the large Kansas City hospitals have purchased land in the county and are intending to build either major health parks or satellite hospitals. One of the two other community hospitals in the area is aggressively moving to shore up its reputation in the part of the county where SMMC had weakest physician response—taking almost the same sequence of steps SMMC had taken 10 years before. The other community hospital, while well regarded, was treading water, stuck in internal political conflict.

The adopted positioning strategy was: We want to maintain and enhance our reputation as the finest hospital in the county. The themeline was: "The pride of Johnson County."

Obvious? Yes. Similar to what many other hospitals might develop as their positioning statements in other markets across the country? Yes. An effective positioning strategy for them? Definitely. Leadership could recognize the elegance of fit to the facts and the promise of additional strength in the marketplace.

Leadership had never thought of themselves quite in this way. The marketplace in effect had reached this conclusion before they had. Their decade-long work had gradually given them this opportunity. Neither had they spoken of themselves in this way. Their messages about themselves went in many different directions.

It was time to strengthen their hard-won position before the big-city competitors arrived and their local competitors could make more strides at their expense.

Once their positioning was clear to themselves, they saw more clearly how to coordinate what they were doing to solidify their position in the market. They also began to talk about themselves in ways that no longer fragmented, but crystallized, their chosen identity.

This was not their only positioning option. They could have positioned themselves in a more distinctive way. They considered, for example, positioning the hospital around wellness.

"We want to be perceived as the hospital most tuned into the staying healthy needs of the community and providing the best wellness programming." As they reflected on that option however, they could see that while it would be distinctive, it wouldn't provide the market with a powerful reason to choose them as a hospital instead of their competitors.

As a hospital, it is first perceived as a place for the care of the sick. That is what all the investments in facilities, staff, and physicians had strengthened and given them a first-class reputation for. The academic discussion that describes health as more than the absence of sickness— true as it is—shouldn't be confused with the way hospitals are perceived: as places where the sick receive care. The hospital that takes on the challenge of changing that very basic perception would take on a very difficult challenge, indeed. It would take on the challenge of not only repositioning the *brand*, in this case Shawnee Mission, it would take on as well the challenge of redefining and repositioning the *product*, namely a hospital.

If they were successful in making the market think of them first and foremost as the wellness provider and not first and foremost as the place to go when sick, they would succeed in placing SMMC in a whole different competitive set, namely, with YMCAs and health clubs. The competitive set would not any longer be hospitals but wellness providers.

Wellness should continue to be part of their mission and an attribute for which they are known, but not their core identity in the mind of the market.

Don't Take a Positioning Strategy That Has Worked Well in One Market and Use It, Without Further Ado, in Another.

Positioning strategies are not transportable. Just because they work in one market does not mean they will work in others.

The best positioning strategies arise through a process similar to that which a physician uses when coming to a definitive diagnosis. It is an *inductive* process rather than a deductive one. A history and physical is taken; all the facts surrounding and leading up to the event are recorded; and the signs, symptoms, and indicators are pieced together one step at a time until the patterns are clear. The term "elegant diagnostician" as used to describe a talented clinician can be ascribed also to a talented marketer developing an effective positioning strategy. The clinician is elegant when she/he picks through the facts, efficiently makes the connections, orders just the right tests—without a barrage of unnecessary effort and expense—and then places her/his finger on just the right diagnosis, one that fits all the facts and leaves nothing unaccounted for. After the diagnosis, which takes so much experience and skill, the prescription is relatively straightforward.

The best positioning strategies too emerge from the facts, they are not superimposed from the outside. Just because something worked elsewhere does not mean it will work here—unless the underlying set of competitive and organizational facts is exactly the same as elsewhere.

Don't Position the Organization as a Whole Without Factoring in the Impact Individual Clinical Services Have on Reputation.

Each clinical service carries its own positioning power and some clinical services have much more of a halo effect than others on the reputation of the hospital as a whole. Clinical services are arranged in terms of their positioning power in a hierarchy.

The service with the greatest ability to influence the market's perception of a hospital is heart services.

The power is so great that when a hospital is rated as the #1 heart hospital, the market often attributes #1 ranking to that hospital for other services—even when the hospital doesn't offer those services.

Second to heart services are neurosurgery and trauma.

These ratings have less to do with healthcare politics or marketing and more to do with anthropology. Simply stated, if your heart or brain waves stop, you're dead. All human song and story celebrate the heart and the mind. Trauma is also a life-and-death type service, so it is grouped by the market near the top of the positioning ladder.

After these three services are arrayed the rest of the clinical services Oncology, for example, has risen on this positioning hierarchy, as more discoveries are made and the more hope the public feels. To the degree that cancer meant death and not *life* and death, it was a service most wanted to ignore.

Orthopedics is also higher on the scale to the degree that it moves away from mere "sawbones" and the more the public is aware of breakthroughs in joint replacements, arthroscopes, human performance labs, and the like.

At the other end of the spectrum are services such as podiatry, proctoscopy, and plastic surgery. Even Shakespeare laughs at feet in Henry V. Again, the ratings are more anthropological than topical. They are not "fair." It can be argued accurately that the health of one's feet is important to the health of the whole body. Nonetheless, being known as the best hospital for podiatry does not contribute mightily to the hospital's overall image and reputation.

It is important, therefore, when developing a positioning strategy to factor in how a given hospital's and competitors' individual clinical services are perceived. Clustered and in combination, certain services will move the reputation in different directions. If, for example, a hospital is recognized for services that deal for the most part with the well— e.g., obstetrics, the not very ill, outpatient surgery—the more the hospital will be perceived as a basic community hospital.

If a hospital is recognized for providing life and death type services— e.g., neonatology, neurosciences, heart services—it will be rated more highly as a place to go when seriously ill and will have more status as a regional draw center.

Selecting, developing, and being recognized for some key service or other can be a legitimate positioning strategy in and of itself. For example, in the North Shore suburbs of Chicago, Evanston Hospital is perceived by the market as the "best" hospital with an excellent medical staff that is university affiliated, has impressive facilities, and is where movers and shakers sit on the board, etc. Nonetheless, in the same community, St. Francis Hospital is recognized as the finest heart hospital, where more open heart surgeries are done than any other in the area. That reputation doesn't displace Evanston Hospital's position as the "best" hospital. It serves St. Francis very well, and *both* are successful.

Steps to Follow in the Development of a Positioning Strategy

Gather and Review the Most Relevant Facts from the Three "Force Fields."

The three "force fields" are: the marketplace's current perception of the hospital and its competitors; the hospital's strengths, limitations, history, and animating values; and what the community thinks of itself and is aspiring towards.

The facts from these three force fields will pull on one another. Taken together they provide a three-dimensional picture of the current situation, where opportunities lie, and what the organization is capable of reaching in a believable way.

The marketplace's current perception of the hospital and its competitors

The first step, therefore, is to map how the hospital is perceived in comparison to competitors on the multiple continua of perception explained in the above section, "High-Tech/High-Touch Is Not the Only Continuum of Perception to Consider When Developing a Positioning Statement" and illustrated in Figures 4-1 through 4-6. The use of both quantitative and qualitative research approaches are recommended.

Most hospitals have already completed a community attitude study that provides much of the objective data required for mapping these perceptions and will have tested how the competitive hospitals are perceived in the continua explained above.

The quantitative research should randomly sample a sufficient number of respondents to be projectable to the population so that leadership has confidence in its accuracy. It will provide a fairly complete, multi-sided view of the competitive situation.

In addition, it makes sense to conduct some qualitative research, either in-depth group interviews (focus groups) or a series of personal interviews with enlightened observers to capture some of the "between the lines" insights about the competitor organizations. Qualitative research gives a more in-depth feel for how things work in a particular market and allows the use of projective techniques. Such between-the-lines insights are frequently the most important insights for developing an effective positioning strategy.

Catherine McAuley Medical Center in Ann Arbor, Michigan, for example, conducted a series of focus groups with key constituents—newspaper writers and editors, community leaders, employees, and key physicians—because they were particularly concerned with whether or not they were "walking as they were talking;" whether their commitment to their mission was recognized by the community; and whether their image coincided with what they were trying to accomplish. They conducted these focus groups in addition to a quantitative study of community attitudes.

Catherine McAuley is a first-rate institution in every sense; and the community does indeed perceive Catherine McAuley as high quality on almost all the perceptual continua. In each of the focus groups, at one time or another, someone would say "whenever anybody is gathered in our community with a healthcare issue or concern, we *expect* a member of Catherine McAuley to be there." Catherine McAuley had established such a high standard for itself that the community had come to expect a very high level of performance and concern. They didn't expect Catherine McAuley to be just any major medical center. They expected Catherine McAuley to make visible a much broader sense of concern for the community's health and well-being. They expected Catherine McAuley to be innovative and responsive to community needs. Those qualities became the touchstone of Catherine McAuley's positioning statement and strategy.

Catherine McAuley's chosen themeline—"Dedicated to making a difference"—expressed this powerfully tenacious commitment in an understated way consistent with its style.

The hospital's strengths, limitations, history, and animating values

After reviewing the first force field, it is usually possible to see the niches that are either unfilled or weakly held by competitors in the marketplace. Before deciding to stake out any particular niche, however, it makes sense that the organization understand its aptitude for staking out that niche. On the one hand, the hospital may overreach itself. The gap between its current image and performance and its chosen positioning may be so great in the mind of the marketplace, that it will not be believed. On the other hand, the positioning may not strike fire within the organization. A positioning needs to be credible not only to the market but also to staff and stakeholders. One hallmark of an effective positioning is that it names the felt identity and aspirations of the organization's staff and rallies them to meet the market more aggressively.

Securing such an understanding of the organization's profile also requires both quantitative and qualitative research.

Quantitative research can be both primary and secondary research. Employee attitude surveys and trend analyses are particularly instructive. Volume trends for each clinical service, market share trends, physician practice trends, financial performance trends, and the history of attempts to target new markets or launch new programs. Completing a comprehensive SWOT (strengths, weaknesses, opportunity, threat analysis) with and through the management and medical staff leadership group is also an important piece of information.

Qualitative research is especially helpful for understanding the genius of an organization, what makes it tick, and the nuances of what makes it special. Hearing key leaders, administrative, medical staff, and board tell their stories, express their dreams, and recount their histories with the organization can be very revealing for a positioning strategy.

Internal trend analysis of Hahnemann University Hospital in Philadelphia, for example, confirmed that Hahnemann was special in the areas of both cancer and heart services. Hahnemann performs the greatest number of open heart surgeries in the Delaware Valley. It has the second strongest cath program and has nationally, if not internationally, recognized leaders in radiation and medical oncology. Its financial performance in the marketplace is strong, especially in comparison to some of the other university hospitals in the market.

It is, however, under-recognized and is not top-of-mind in the Philadelphia marketplace.

Qualitative research provides additional insight into Hahnemann's identity and the touchstone for an effective positioning strategy. Hahnemann's clinical faculty members, while not as a whole renowned for basic research, are very proficient in translating the latest to the bedside. A number of clinical chiefs are very proficient at translating theory into practice. They practice with an entrepreneurial, energetic style. Therefore, Hahnemann's positioning is: "the hospital that quickly brings the latest discoveries in medicine to the bedside." Its themeline struck a recognizable chord in employees and clinical leadership as well as the marketplace: "Discover Hahnemann Healing."

What the community thinks of itself and is aspiring towards

This third force field will also heavily influence the choice of the positioning strategy. If review of the first force field reveals where the closed, open, and weakly held niches in the mind of the market are, and review of the second force field reveals what's special and appropriate for the hospital, review of the third force field reveals what's special about the market—in terms of underlying values, unmet needs, and current developments.

A combination of quantitative and qualitative research is appropriate for exploring this force field as well. A review of demographic trends, business formation and employment trends, attitudinal research concerning perceived quality of life, and future prospects provides an introductory understanding of a given community.

Following up the quantitative analysis with in-depth probing of knowledgeable community leaders through focus groups or personal interviews provides a much deeper understanding of a particular marketplace. Some fruitful areas to probe: history and turning points in the life of the community; preferred cultural values or style of the community, institutions, or people that are admired in the community; local political and religious trends and values; current important events or brouhahas; a review of who are the in and active groups in the community and why; and a review of how attitudes toward local hospitals have developed over time.

For example, when developing a positioning and a new name for two merged hospitals in Corona, California, it was important to combine insights from all three force fields.

The mapping of community perceptions of competitive healthcare providers on the various continua of comparison revealed that the two hospitals were perceived similarly, as basic community hospitals, and that a third hospital on the edge of the service area was beginning to intrude and had the mind share to capitalize in terms of additional market share.

A review of the strengths and attitudes of the new leadership of the combined hospital revealed a commitment to growth, given the combining of resources, and a desire to wipe the slate completely clean of past rivalries and identities.

Review of community trends showed a still burgeoning community in terms of jobs, new business formation, and a much larger population base within a few short years—up to much more than 100,000 population in the immediate service area, and 250,000 in the combined primary and secondary service areas. Probing what was happening in the community revealed the following:

- Strong, mutually exclusive loyalties to each hospital by equal size segments of the longer term residents.

- Some schizophrenia in the community between long-established residents who had roots in the "citrus capital of the world" and newer residents—mainly Orange County ex-patriates who still kept their loyalties to Orange County—driving back there for work, shopping, *and* their healthcare needs.

- A "second city" mentality to Orange County.

- An underlying desire for first rate institutions to anchor the community.

Given the intense attachments of one-half of the community to the two previous institutions, it made sense in the name and positioning to not erase all relations with the past. Given the unfolding shape of the previously schizophrenic community, it made sense to position the merged hospitals as the harbinger of the coming together of the community. Given what the growing community was longing for and the market demand arising from a growing population, it made sense to position the new entity as a major player.

Therefore, the new name of the combined Circle City Medical Center and Corona Community Hospital became Corona Regional Medical Center.

Name: Corona Regional Medical Center

Corona because that's the name of the large, growing, attractive community that is the hub of the service area. *Regional* because some of the combined hospital's services will have a regional draw, because the combined institution has much more strength than the two individual hospitals had had separately, and because the hospital would be serving an even larger service area than Corona. *Medical Center* because the new institution has two operating campuses. One hospital was renamed "Main Hospital" because that's where the medical/surgical, obstetric, and emergency services are located (it also happens to be on Main Street); and the other serves as the Rehabilitation Hospital, where the physical medicine and rehab and mental health rehab services are located.

Themeline: Partners in Health and Healing

This has multiple meanings. It refers to the coming together of institutions as a harbinger of the community's coming together. It refers to the style of practice preferred by younger families looking for a partnership relationship with their healthcare providers. It expresses the desire of employers for cooperative arrangements. And it relates to the desire of physicians in the region to be treated with respect and collaboration by the newly emerging, more powerful than ever hospital.

Without an in-depth understanding of the community's history and hopes, the positioning would not have been as on target strategically. (See Exhibit 4-2)

A fresh contemporary mark that expresses a new beginning and depicts visually the pulling together of disparate elements. The mark can be seen as a crown (the English translation of the Latin "Corona") and as a sheaf, reflecting the rural, farming roots of the community.

Exhibit 4-1: Corona Regional Medical Center

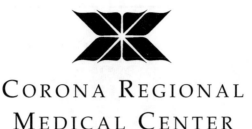

CORONA REGIONAL
MEDICAL CENTER

Partners in Health and Healing.

Condense the Most Relevant Facts from the Three Force Fields into One List—One to Two Pages Long.

The facts from the three force fields should pull on one another. Before deciding on the final positioning strategy, experiment with some hypotheses based on different key facts in the summary statement to see if they do justice to all the key facts—much as a clinician's diagnosis has to "explain" or fit all the relevant facts.

Take, for example, the following summary of facts from the three force fields surrounding an osteopathic hospital on one of the coasts:

1) The hospital serves as the training site for all new osteopaths from a multi-state region.

2) All the specialists on staff are perceived as superb by the primary-care physicians on staff: They'd say "cardiology, excellent," "pathology, excellent," "orthopedics, excellent" and so on.

3) The hospital is located in an attractive, upper middle class neighborhood.

4) It is housed in a one-story building that gives the impression of a second-rate motel.

5) Most of the DOs on staff practice at other MD hospitals, but not vice versa.

6) The younger DOs in particular lament "nobody knows what we are."

Exhibit 4-2: Corona Regional Medical Center's "Partners in Health and Healing"

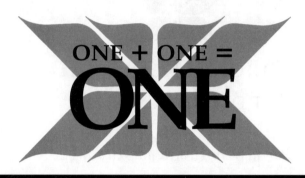

ONE + ONE = ONE

INTRODUCING

CORONA REGIONAL MEDICAL CENTER
Partners in Health and Healing.

The equation is simple, but the sum more significant than it seems. This is the result when committed people build on common strengths to forge a bright and better future. Corona Community Hospital and Circle City Medical Center have come together to form a stronger, more vital health care resource for our community and the region.

ONE + ONE = EXCEPTIONAL HEALTH CARE

Corona Regional Medical Center unites the qualities of two respected institutions to bring forward the best facilities, the latest technology and experienced physicians and staff. It is a bold and promising step forward.

✖ Remodeling will rejuvenate both facilities and make each ready for specialized services. The former Corona Community will be renamed Corona Regional Medical Center – Main Hospital, where patient services such as the new obstetrics unit, surgery, and the intensive care unit, to name a few, will be offered. Circle City will be renamed Corona Regional Medical Center – Rehabilitation Hospital, a facility devoted to the special needs of rehabilitation and psychiatric patients, opening in the spring. In the coming weeks, we'll detail the services provided at each facility.

✖ By the end of November, all emergencies will be cared for at Corona Regional Medical Center – Main Hospital, 800 South Main Street in Corona.

✖ Staff physicians at both hospitals will continue to care for their patients at the new Corona Regional Medical Center.

✖ All insurance plans currently accepted at both hospitals will be honored by the new Corona Regional Medical Center.

✖ A special information "Answer Line" has been set up to take your questions. Just Call 714.736.7272

ONE + ONE = CORONA REGIONAL MEDICAL CENTER
Partners in Health and Healing.

CORONA REGIONAL
MEDICAL CENTER

MAIN HOSPITAL, 800 South Main Street, Corona 91720 714.737.4343
REHABILITATION HOSPITAL, 730 Magnolia Avenue, Corona 91719 714.735.1211

Corona Regional Medical Center does not discriminate on the basis of sex, race, religion, color, national origin, handicap or age.

INTRODUCING

A NEW PARTNERSHIP OF

HEALTH, HEALING... AND VISION.

CORONA

REGIONAL

MEDICAL

CENTER

You can sense it growing all over Corona. It's an energy you can actually feel; a vitality you can almost touch. It's a new optimism encouraging us to work together to build on the strengths of yesterday to create a bright new future of growth and prosperity. Not just for our city, but for the entire inland region.

As in any community on the verge of rapid growth, one of our most pressing needs is for a strong, comprehensive medical resource. An institution able to serve the increased health and healing needs of our community, with the resources – and the vision – to keep pace with the community as it grows.

Introducing Corona Regional Medical Center.

From two long-respected institutions, Corona Community Hospital and Circle City Medical Center, we have forged a new medical resource greater than the sum of its parts. Corona Regional Medical Center is the consolidation of progressive facilities, leading-edge technology and highly-experienced medical professionals and specialists into a single medical center every resident of our city – and our region – can depend on. Today, tomorrow and well beyond.

All of us at Corona Regional Medical Center are excited about the prospect of serving our long-time friends even better, and of making friendships with new members of our community as they discover the advanced care and resources of our new institution.

CORONA REGIONAL MEDICAL CENTER
Partners in Health and Healing.

800 South Main Street Corona, California 91720   714.737.4343
730 Magnolia Avenue Corona, California 91719   714.735.1211

7) Chiropractic is by far the fastest growing healthcare-related service in the area.

8) The older DOs still do manipulation and are very busy.

9) The hospital has low top-of-mind awareness and name recognition ratings in its local community compared to competitive hospitals.

The hospital was in a downward spiral and recognized that it needed to stake out a strong position and then consistently work to reinforce it. As various members of leadership reviewed these facts, they differed on which facts were most suggestive of a positioning strategy. Some of the options suggested:

- From facts #1 and #2: Position the hospital in terms of its training program and its specialists.

- From facts #2 and #6: Position the hospital and the osteopaths "as good as MDs" and do a public education campaign on the DOs' extensive training program that is equivalent to what an MD receives.

- From fact #4: Most wanted to address the facility issue but recognize that as a tactic and not a positioning strategy.

- From facts #3 and #9: Position the hospital as a convenient, community resource. The positioning actually utilized by the hospital and featured in all its collateral was "friendly neighbor." It obviously hadn't worked.

- From facts #7 and #8: The best positioning strategy emerged, namely to position the hospital and osteopaths not as "everything an MD is" but as "everything an MD is and more." The strength of this positioning as opposed to the others: it tunes into the large part of the market that goes underserved and dissatisfied and that is looking for more than traditional medicine gives them. Instead of trying to be merely equal to the MD, feature the fact that osteopathy is "hands on." Celebrate the tradition of manipulation and take pride in it. It is precisely what a sizeable segment is looking for and the direction in which the market as a whole is heading.

The drawbacks of the first positioning: specialist excellence and training site status. It was "me too" in nature. It staked out a niche already strongly occupied by competitors. It added one more voice singing the same song. It made it that much more difficult to be heard.

The second positioning, "equal to an MD," was critiqued as an also-ran, wannabe, imitation positioning. It declared the osteopath as never quite the real thing because it accepted the MD as the standard of comparison.

Subject the Alternative Positionings Emerging from the Force Field Analysis to the Threefold Test.

1) Does the positioning stake out a niche that is empty or weakly held—i.e., the current occupant can be displaced and it won't take a resource investment that will bankrupt the organization?

2) Does the positioning strike chords internally and stimulate pride? It is alright if it leaves room for growth. The organization may not yet fill out the niche fully, and it may still be on the way to full stature—but nonetheless it recognizes itself in the positioning.

3) It names something important to the marketplace, a value that will give it pause and reason to choose the organization over competitors—in and of itself or all things being equal.

Using this critique on the final option suggested in the exercise above reveals:

• The positioning "all that traditional medical care offers and more" stakes out a niche no other hospital holds.

• The positioning expresses values that are strongly held by staff members and carries forward the organization's history and traditions.

• The positioning corresponds to a value for which a large part of the market is searching.

Positioning: Emblazoning a Chosen Positioning on the Mind of the Marketplace

Once a chosen positioning is selected, the challenge is then to move the market from the image that it currently has of the hospital to the desired image or positioning that has been chosen. Recognizing that the market is slow to change once it has made up its mind, and recognizing all the clutter in the channels of communication, it will be important to aggressively wield the four tools of repositioning at one's command. The positioning strategy is no more than mumbling to oneself if it isn't taken aggressively to market. The four tools are:

1) The power of word-of-mouth networks

2) The power of the internal market

3) The power of symbolic actions: bold moves and fine touches

4) The power of integrated communications campaigns

A repositioning plan of action will typically utilize all four tools but in varying degrees of emphasis, depending on the situation and the positioning.

The Power of Word-of-Mouth Networks

The first tool is to organize the power of word-of-mouth networks. This approach combines communication theory, which traces how messages pass into a culture from opinion leaders through their networks and from elites to the multitudes, with the principles of community organizing.

Mobilizing word-of-mouth networks is a communications tool that is almost uniquely available to a hospital. Very few organizations have staff persons, for example, with the title of director of community relations. Hospitals can take such a proactive role because they are large, local organizations whose missions are perceived as beneficent and important for all members of the community—cutting across age, sex, ethnic, income, or religious identities. It is a shame, therefore, that more hospitals don't fully utilize their community relations/building/organizing potential.

Saul Alinsky, the dean and theorist of contemporary community organizing, has much to teach the healthcare marketer.

- Work with the "intermediate structures," the voluntary associations within the community that already are organized, have a reason to meet in an ongoing way, and are in face-to-face communication.

- Identify an issue that has such felt importance that the group can be rallied around it.

- Work with the natural leaders, as opposed to the titular leaders, of the group to frame the issue.

- Provide the group a way to take *action* on the issue—to free them from the pain of talking an issue to death and from "meeting-itis."

Examples of hospitals using these approaches:

One hospital worked with the natural leaders of women's groups in the area to identify issues of importance and organize an action response. Out of their work arose a prenatal care clinic for disadvantaged expectant mothers, which received broad financial and volunteer community support and dramatically reduced infant mortality and morbidity.

This collaborative effort brought a whole range of influential women into close contact with the hospital. Its message, aspirations, and positioning were shared in person and up close—not as the central point on their agenda together, but as part of the getting to know one another.

Another hospital worked with a range of community senior groups. Out of their collaboration developed a day care program for older adults that received broad community support. By and by, the hospital was much better known and recognized by these leaders and by their constituents.

The community organizing approach takes community relations one step further. If the aim of community relations is to keep community groups satisfied with the hospital, the aim of community organizing is to see them mobilized. If the aim of community relations is cordial community feelings, the aim of community organizing is collaborative community action.

The Power of the Internal Market

Mobilize the power of the internal market. Employees, volunteers, board members, physicians, and their spouses are a potentially "megahertz" communication channel.

Internal stakeholders, for example, are important sources of direct referrals. Any intelligent marketing plan for a particular service starts by making sure that staff nurses are well-informed and hopefully very impressed by the quality of a service. Many people looking for a particular type of a physician ask the nurses they know. Many people researching the quality of a service or a physician ask nurses as an integral part of that research. Nurses known by their neighbors, friends, and acquaintances for working in a hospital obstetrics unit, for example, have the power in many situations of making or breaking an obstetrician's practice. Nurses are thought to be an objective, knowledgeable, user-friendly reference source.

Moreover, without extra effort, there is often little horizontal, cross-service communication. What is prized and valued by one department is often faintly understood or recognized by others.

It makes sense, therefore, to start a repositioning campaign with the internal stakeholders. They represent hundreds, and in a large hospital even thousands, of potential salespersons in the community. They in turn are trusted information and opinion resources for many others. One hospital in Wisconsin, for example, wondered why it was seeing an upsurge in business from a community 20 miles away and well outside of its traditional service area. The increase was traced to the pediatric head nurse who lived in that community. She was constantly talking up that hospital and its physicians to her friends and neighbors.

It has often happened that a hospital has launched a communications campaign to the media without first explaining and previewing the campaign with staff members and auxiliary within. In that situation it has been known to happen that a neighbor of an employee will come up to her/him saying "I saw your ad"—because for her/his neighbors the employee represents or embodies the organization. It is a downer for that employee when that employee has to say to her/himself and to the neighbor, "What ad?" At that moment the employee doesn't feel that she/he represents the hospital, instead she/he feels discounted by and unimportant to her/his employer.

Imagine instead the hospital that takes the time to preview a repositioning strategy and campaign with the employees and the other supporters and stakeholders of the hospital. Imagine the hospital explaining the facts and challenge behind the strategy, providing an in-depth rationale for the strategy, inviting suggestions, and enlisting employee support. Imagine the employee in that scenario who is approached by the neighbor saying "I saw your ad." At that point, the employee, empowered with facts and fully informed, will be able to say "yes, and let me tell you more" amplifying and intensifying the campaign's effect in the marketplace. Imagine all 100, 1,000, 4,000 employees as active salespersons in their communities.

That approach is precisely the approach Hahnemann University Hospital took before launching its major television campaign. The commercials featured its leading-edge cancer and heart services and ended with a call to action and the tag line, "Discover Hahnemann Healing." Before the campaign was launched, each employee received a direct-mail piece from the president of the university saying, "You are about to be discovered." The piece gave visual excerpts from the commercials, articulated the strategy behind them, and provided the facts that substantiate the heart and cancer services as among the finest in the area. (See Exhibit 4-3.)

Moreover, the hospital conducted an internal launch featuring a videotape of live glimpses of employees and physicians practicing "Hahnemann Healing;" a continuous-loop, advance showing of the commercials; and a kick-off rally in the cafeteria where visible expressions of the theme line were distributed to employees—from fanny packs and mugs, to banners and pens. "Discover Hahnemann Healing" was established within the organization before it was communicated to others. The employees were empowered to support and amplify the message in the media with their networks of friends and neighbors.

The Power of Symbolic Actions: Bold Moves and Fine Touches

Use the power of symbolic actions. It is a truism that actions speak louder than words. Words may express lofty sentiments, noble ideals, and good intentions, but still be empty. It is one thing to talk. It is another thing to walk the talk. The marketplace will be intrigued by words, but it will not be convinced until it sees the behavior. Actions express identity much more effectively than words alone.

Moreover, some actions are much more convincing than other actions. Some actions have the power to break through the clutter, capture attention, and clearly present one's chosen identity even without benefit of interpretive words.

Actions with these attributes are called **symbolic actions** because they dip into the natural communicative power of symbols. Consider how symbols work.

A Message from Iphid E. Bares, President and Chief Executive Officer, Hahnemann University

Hahnemann University is a leading academic health center, and you are the reason why. It is your experience, your professionalism, your dedication and your caring that keep us on the leading edge of medicine and health education. And now we believe it's time Philadelphia—and the whole Delaware Valley—learned more about you and Hahnemann... and about our many accomplishments.

That's why we've decided to launch a new full-scale advertising and public relations campaign. Our goal is to inform our community of all of the leading-edge services Hahnemann University provides, and of the special kind of medicine that sets us apart as educators, health-care providers, and researchers.

So take a few minutes to read this short piece and find out a little bit more about our new campaign and all its elements. It is, after all, about you.

Hahnemann University's New Advertising Campaign Is Designed To Tell Our Community Just How Televised and Successful You Are.

Television Our advertising campaign's two major components will be a pair of 30-second television commercials that will focus on Hahnemann's expertise in cancer and in cardiac care. ■ The new spots will highlight Hahnemann's exceptional record of success with even the most difficult heart and cancer cases. To help us make the point as powerfully as possible, we'll be using footage of a number of famous Philadelphia sports teams that overcame long odds, and won championships. ■ The first spot tells the story of Hahnemann's expertise in cancer treatment, and uses film of the Philadelphia Eagles, and of our friends (and dedicated supporters of the Hahnemann bone marrow transplant program) the Philadelphia Flyers, during their 1974 and 1975 Stanley Cup Championship seasons. The second commercial features the Likoff Cardiovascular Institute and cardiac surgery, and will use footage of the 1980 Major League Baseball Champion Philadelphia Phillies, and the 1983 NBA Champion Philadelphia 76ers. ■

Combining film and tape of these famous sports teams with dramatic footage shot at Hahnemann University, our commercials document and celebrate the "winning moment" in sports... and in Hahnemann healing.

Print Ads The second component of the Hahnemann University advertising campaign will be a series of full-page print advertisements which will appear in the Sunday *Philadelphia Inquirer* magazine. Like our television commercial, our print ads will concentrate on communicating the story of Hahnemann's exceptional record in treating and curing the toughest kinds of medical problems. ■ The focus of our first print advertisements will also be on cancer and cardiac care.

Public Relations In addition to our television advertising, we will be mounting a multi-faceted public relations campaign which will help keep Hahnemann University in the minds of our community year-round. ■ Our first event will be a very special one. In conjunction with the American Cancer Society, Hahnemann is sponsoring Breast Cancer Awareness Month in May. The highlight of the series of screening and education programs will be "A Conversation with Ann Jillian."

The three-time Emmy nominee and Golden Globe Award-winning actress is one of Hollywood's best-known survivors of breast cancer. Ms. Jillian is renowned as one of the finest speakers on the subject, presenting a positive and hopeful message that has already helped women all over the country take control of their breast health. The date of Ms. Jillian's address is Saturday, May 2. ■ In addition, during the first two weeks of May, Hahnemann will be offering free breast screenings, and reduced-price mammograms to women who qualify. ■ Our Breast Cancer Awareness program is one of a number of special events we will sponsor this year.

The Delaware Valley Is About To

DISCOVER HAHNEMANN HEALING.

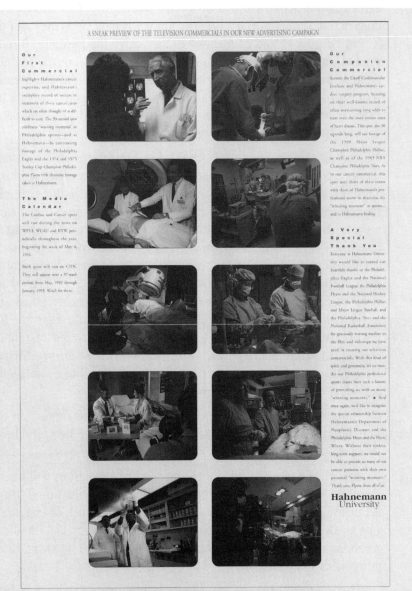

Symbols go well beyond words in their expressive power because, unlike words, symbols already partake in what they point to. Words are "conventional" signs, meaning what they do because human beings agree that particular clusters of sounds will signify X. Symbols, on the other hand, signify not just because human beings agree they will mean X, but because in and of themselves they carry the meaning. A natural symbol such as the north star, for example, stands for constancy not just because human beings have arbitrarily agreed it should, but because it stands predictably in the skies allowing human beings to navigate by its light. Human gestures such as an outreached hand are symbols that carry meaning even without words.

Consider, for example, a hospital that positions itself as a four-star service organization. How does it best communicate that positioning? Through actions that speak with the power of symbols. For example, at Phoebe Putney Memorial Hospital in Albany, Georgia, if patients or visitors choose not to use the hospital's valet service and instead park their own cars, they are greeted as they emerge from their cars by a smiling young man wearing a red blazer and driving a white golf cart with "From Phoebe with Love" written on the side. He warmly welcomes all, piles them and their belongings into the cart, whisks them to the front door, helps them alight, and hands them over to the inside advisors who make sure they have clear instructions and assistance, if needed, to arrive easily at their destinations. Phoebe Putney Memorial Hospital is perceived to walk the talk. With these and other symbolic actions it conveys its chosen positioning.

Some actions are able at one and the same time to capture an intention, unerringly search out the sensibilities of the customers, and light up that meaning before their eyes.

Some leaders have a gift for recognizing which actions will have this threefold power. They know how to convey their intentions through actions that have just the right spin, surprise, and touch of imagination. Just as an actor with good timing and the right gesture can illuminate a scene, so also some leaders act and the market notices. In short, they are gifted with symbol mastery.

These actions can take the form of **bold moves**, which are writ large and generate attention from a broad audience. For example, a CEO trying to reposition his hospital from a sleepy, passive organization into one that is aggressive and on the move purchased a vacant piece of land across from a competitive hospital and placed a sign on the property saying "future home of the Outpatient Surgery Center" of his Hospital. He caused heads to turn and rivers of editorial ink and letters to the editor to flow.

Another CEO, who had secured a large grant from a very prominent local citizen, began construction of a major comprehensive cancer center—to be named after that most prominent citizen's wife—just weeks before a competitive hospital was to announce its plans for a similar project.

Or the symbol mastery can express itself in **fine touches** that dramatize the positioning no less tellingly but on a smaller scale—as when a CEO changed the disposable plates on patient trays to china plates and who threw out the old, see-through, postage-stamp-size towels in the patient bathrooms and purchased large, logo-bearing, fluffy new towels from the same source as the Ritz-Carlton hotel chain. Patients and staff began to recognize the patient-centered positioning without ever hearing or reading a word.

It is not always necessary to develop a whole new set of actions as part of the repositioning plan. Sometimes what a hospital is already planning to do will convey the positioning to the market. Because the positioning strategy has been clarified, planned actions can be better coordinated and timed for maximum impact.

Shawnee Mission Medical Center, for example, was already planning to recruit a new, well-regarded cardiac surgeon to its staff and sponsor—with one of its surgeons who has a national reputation for innovative laparoscopy applications—a national symposium for surgeons on laparoscopic advances.

Leadership realized that those actions not only served their own discrete ends, they also helped strengthen and convey the positioning strategy "Leading hospital in Johnson County."

Using the Quality Hospital matrix as a guide, they were able to see how physician recruitment and a national symposium not only rooted the positioning more firmly in reality, but helped, with appropriate publicity, convey the positioning to the public.

Some other actions, designed to maintain or improve the public's perception and rating on selected continua of quality, were selected for implementation and publicity.

- Already perceived as providing the finest nursing care in the area, leadership decided to maintain its current, rather rich nurse-to-patient ratios and expand its innovative nursing staff development program.

- Given the growing perception of the hospital as a leader *(noblesse oblige)*, management recommitted to its extensive Wellness program for the benefit of the community and planned to expand its well attended and regarded Thanksgiving Day community celebration.

- Leadership recognized, moreover, what some of its "fine touches" were doing for the hospital's reputation. The public was well aware of and impressed by the hospital's tradition of landscaping. Grand beds of seasonal flowers, kept lovingly at the entrances to the hospital, impressed and delighted the eyes of all who saw them. Flowers lovingly maintained bespoke a hospital that shows care to the point of beauty.

The Power of Integrated Communications Campaigns

Use the power of integrated marketing communications to implement a successful positioning campaign. Therefore, it makes sense to follow these five guidelines:

1) Devote sufficient resources to the campaign.

2) Make sure it is a campaign, not spotty promotions.

3) Focus in the campaign on the elements with the greatest intrinsic positioning power.

4) Coordinate appropriate service-specific campaigns as subsets of the positioning campaign, and design them to achieve image enhancement as well as business development objectives.

5) Plan and execute public relations and paid advertising together so they feed on one another and multiply the reach and frequency of the campaign.

Devote Sufficient Resources to the Campaign.

Devote sufficient resources to the campaign to make it worthwhile. This guideline relates to the objectives of the campaign and the methods used to track its effectiveness.

At the very least, the positioning campaign should aim to achieve three objectives:

1) The campaign should produce a substantial uptick on the market's rating of the hospital on the variable selected as the key to the positioning strategy.

   For example, if a hospital chose as its positioning strategy, "We want to be perceived as the hospital most tuned in to the needs of women," the hospital would first need a baseline measure of where it currently stands, e.g., "Currently 15 percent of the market perceives our hospital as the hospital most tuned in to the needs of women." The objective of the campaign will be to see X increase in the percentage of the market that has not only heard and understood the message, but that is also convinced and able to describe the hospital in synch with its chosen positioning.

   What increase is it feasible to project and in what period of time? It depends on four variables—how cluttered the channels of communication are; whether competitors will be further clogging the channels with a message that will confuse or dilute the message; what resources are put into the campaign and how efficiently they are used to produce adequate reach and frequency in the target audience; and finally, the attention grabbing power of what is said and done to communicate the message.

   The decision concerning how high to aim—i.e., what percentage increase in the target audience to expect—emerges from an analysis of how much *thrust* will be put into the campaign against how much *resistance* that thrust will meet. If the channels of communication are cluttered and the market starts from an attitude of indifference or negativity towards the hospital, the greater the thrust required. The thrust is both energy and mass—dynamism of the message is the energy, and the frequency and reach of exposure to the message is the mass.

In a rural community, for example, fewer resources will typically be required to communicate a message because the word-of-mouth networks are so strong and the channels of communication less cluttered. In a major urban market, a greater resource investment will be required. If the repositioning campaign is to be more than wishful thinking, enough resources need to be devoted to it to reach the anticipated changes in the market's perception.

2) A second measure of a positioning campaign's effectiveness is the percent of the market able to associate the theme line with the sponsoring hospital.

The themeline is meant to be a distillation of the positioning strategy in a memorable form. It makes sense, therefore, to expect that it will be remembered and associated with the hospital. This measure also serves as a measure of the quality of the creative work and of the way the theme line is applied and utilized.

3) The third measure of a positioning campaign's effectiveness is the change in the market's level of *preference* for the hospital. The angle of identity presented to the marketplace through the positioning should be valued enough by the market to influence its intention to use the hospital. In this way, the positioning campaign goes beyond mere image management. It is designed to form an image in the market's mind that will cause it to *prefer* the hospital over competitors. Image clarification that influences preference.

Make Sure It Is a Campaign, Not Spotty Promotions.

It is estimated that it takes six to eight exposures for a target audience even to notice a given message. Just when the sponsor of a communication is beginning to tire of a message, the market is just noticing it. Effective communication therefore depends on intelligent repetition.

A one-shot ad or spotty promotion could just as well be left undone because it is effort and money down the drain.

To think campaign is to develop the appropriate communications mix and media schedule that will provide multiple ways of reaching the target audience—a poster message here, a community presentation there, a radio reminder here, a print execution there—until a sizeable portion of the market has been reached and the message registered.

Focus in the Campaign on the Elements with the Greatest Intrinsic Positioning Power.

Those symbolic actions or services that best convey the positioning receive first attention from communications in the positioning campaign.

Mercy/St. Mary's Health Services in Grand Rapids, Michigan, for example, positioning itself as the "harbinger of the next generation of healthcare delivery" focused on its strengths in primary care; its critical path initiatives that were producing real savings through physician/hospital cooperation; its case management; and its caring for patients in the most appropriate settings down the line from inpatient care—outpatient, SNF, home care its prevention and health maintenance initiatives. The system had put together the package that prepared it for the coming capitated, competing healthcare delivery system era.

Among the elements of the positioning campaign that received promotion dollars and support, the campaign dramatized the role of the primary-care physician as the patients' health advocate and quarterback through the sickness care system.

Why? The primary-care physician will be key in the coming era and embodies the skills and approaches that will be valued.

The campaign also selected for special attention through public relations the story of its Clinica Santa Maria, a free OB clinic for pregnant teenagers designed to provide adequate prenatal care. The story emphasized how much money the clinic had saved the healthcare system. Most young women who had not received adequate prenatal care in the past were receiving it. The number of premature babies delivered by young mothers in the area had dropped dramatically. The number of babies admitted to neonatology was down proportionately. The bill to society for neonatology services was down just as dramatically. The clinic no doubt demonstrated the hospital's commitment to the poor. Just as clearly, it embodied the hospital's efforts to bring down society's healthcare bill—the harbinger of the coming healthcare delivery era.

Coordinate Appropriate Service-Specific Campaigns as Subsets of the Positioning Campaign, and Design Them to Achieve Image Enhancement as Well as Business Development Objectives.

The debate whether a hospital should do image campaigns or service-specific campaigns is a false debate and dichotomy. It is important to build brand equity. Strong brand equity supports all the services and all the doctors on staff. Service-specific campaigns, depending on the positioning chosen, can carry the positioning strategy into the market.

Consider, for example, the following four specific television commercials for four different services at Clarkson Hospital. Each of them ends with the themeline—"another first from Clarkson Hospital," reinforcing Clarkson's positioning as the first in the double sense of oldest and leading.

It wasn't necessary for Clarkson to do more than these service specific ads to convey its positioning strategy. But by planning and executing them in a coordinated way, Clarkson was able to establish its positioning in the mind of the marketplace. Both business development and image enhancement objectives were met. (See Exhibit 4-4.)

Plan and Execute Public Relations and Paid Advertising Together So They Feed on One Another and Multiply the Reach and Frequency of the Campaign.

Any split or rivalry between public relations and paid advertising is only in the mind of its professional practitioners. There are two very powerful complementary ways to tell the hospital's story, and should be integrated as a double-barreled shotgun that doubles the volume of the shots expelled, and widens the target reached.

With paid advertising, the message sent is what the hospital crafts and the setting for the message is what the hospital chooses. In brief, the advantages of paid advertising are control over message and medium. The drawbacks of paid advertising are, however, that the organization is blowing its own horn rather than an objective, credible outside party; and secondly, it is costly.

With public relations, the hospital's message is communicated by an outside, objective third party. It is not the hospital blowing its own horn, it is the editor, the anchor person, the reporter. It is therefore more believable. Moreover, it is free—except for the time of the staff person

Exhibit 4-4: Clarkson Hospital's Commercial Storyboards

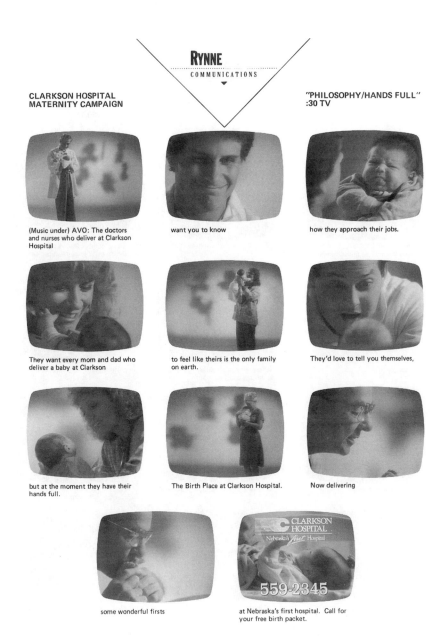

CLARKSON HOSPITAL MATERNITY CAMPAIGN

RYNNE COMMUNICATIONS

"PHILOSOPHY/HANDS FULL" :30 TV

(Music under) AVO: The doctors and nurses who deliver at Clarkson Hospital

want you to know

how they approach their jobs.

They want every mom and dad who deliver a baby at Clarkson

to feel like theirs is the only family on earth.

They'd love to tell you themselves,

but at the moment they have their hands full.

The Birth Place at Clarkson Hospital.

Now delivering

some wonderful firsts

at Nebraska's first hospital. Call for your free birth packet.

Exhibit 4-4: Clarkson Hospital's Commercial Storyboards (continued)

**CLARKSON HOSPITAL
HEART POSITIONING**

**"FIRST IN HEARTS"
:30 TV**

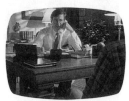

(Music under) DOCTOR: Well, I know you've had success with this procedure . . .

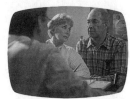

AVO: There's a hospital in Omaha

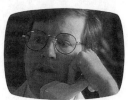

where doctors from a five-state region send their heart patients.

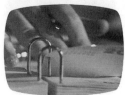

A hospital

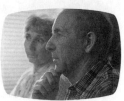

where an extraordinary group of heart specialists

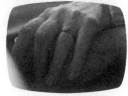

perform more heart procedures

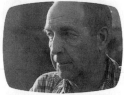

than anywhere else in Omaha.

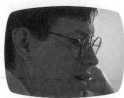

Whose specialists have pioneered

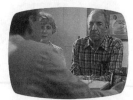

many state firsts—including the first cardiac catheterization

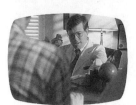

and heart transplant.

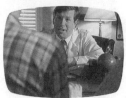

DOCTOR: You're set for Clarkson on Wednesday.

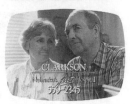

AVO: Cardiac Care at Clarkson Hospital. It's why we're first in the hearts of many.

Exhibit 4-4: Clarkson Hospital's Commercial Storyboards (continued)

RYNNE
COMMUNICATIONS

CLARKSON HOSPITAL
ONCOLOGY CAMPAIGN

"TWO HEADS"
:30 TV

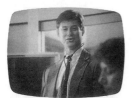

DR. SCHUE: Morning, Alicia.

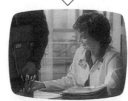

AVO: There's a committee that meets weekly.

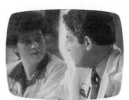

It consists of some of the brightest, most dedicated people in Omaha.
DR. THOMPSON: Good weekend?

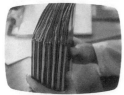

AVO: It's not a social group.

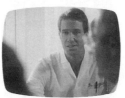

DR. KINGSTON: Let's get started.

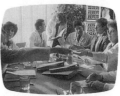

AVO: It's the Clarkson Cancer team.

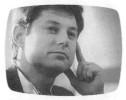

Specialists who review the progress of each cancer patient

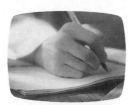

being treated at Clarkson Hospital.

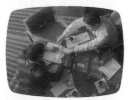

Because if two heads are better than one,

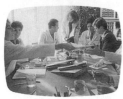

why stop at two?

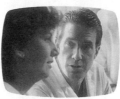

DR. KINGSTON: Good plan! Let's go on to the next patient.

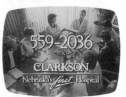

AVO: Coordinated Cancer Care. Call Clarkson Hospital. Another first from Nebraska's first hospital.

Upgrading a Hospital's Image   **179**

Exhibit 4-4: Clarkson Hospital's Commercial Storyboards (continued)

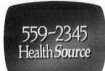

**CLARKSON HOSPITAL
PHYSICIAN REFERRAL**

RYNNE
C O M M U N I C A T I O N S

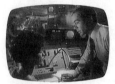

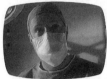

**"DOCTOR/PATIENT"
:30 TV**

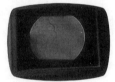

(Music under) AVO: This is the number to call

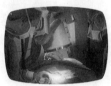

to reach doctors known for their

exceptional medical expertise.

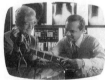

(MUSIC)

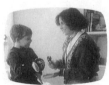

(MUSIC)

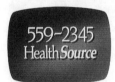

This is also the number to call

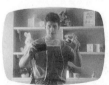

to reach doctors known for

their exceptional care.

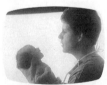

Doctors whose first priority is always you. Whatever your medical need.

To find a doctor like this,

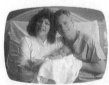

call HealthSource,

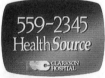

559-2345. A service of Clarkson Hospital.

who, unseen or heard, has worked to fashion and place the story. Finally, a good story can multiply itself and cascade in ever widening circles. A local story may catch regional interest, may be picked up by the wires, go national, and then double back into regional and local features.

On the other hand, with public relations, the message cannot be controlled. The reporter may give the story a negative spin or may turn the message every which way, but loose. Secondly, the timing of the story is not controlled. The story may break at an inconvenient, complicating, or opportune time—one never knows for sure. Finally, where and how the story appears isn't controlled. It may appear in the gossip, financial, or current events sections. It may appear over, under, or next to stories about competitors, axe murderers, or papal visits. The risks of aggressive public relations, however, can usually be managed and pale in comparison to potential rewards.

Each time a paid ad is developed, it should be done with an eye to its public relations potential.

Consider, for example, the storyboard for Clarkson's Over 50 Club. Cast for the lead in the television commercial was a 70-year-old actor in superb physical condition. He beat out his 50-year-old son for the part. Not only was he an expert diver and all around athlete, he and his wife were award-winning ballroom dancers. He exemplified what a healthy lifestyle for seniors was all about. (See Exhibit 4-5.)

The public relations professionals saw the potential news value in this story. He was taken on a media tour at the same time as the ad campaign was launched. He appeared on every news program in town. Some of the news programs aired "gratis" parts of the Clarkson ad as the lead into his interview. The total time for each showing of the ad: 30 seconds. The total air time as a result of the public relations initiative: 60 full minutes. Moreover, the air time was free and in a credible news program context.

Public relations and paid advertising can be planned and executed in a way that corrects the limits of each and so that each leverages the impact of the other.

Any positioning campaign that uses only paid advertising without integrating public relations as well—or vice versa—is only fractionally effective in comparison to a campaign that integrates the two.

Exhibit 4-5: Clarkson Hospital's "Health and Wellness Club" Commercial Storyboard

**CLARKSON HOSPITAL
HEALTH AND WELLNESS CLUB**

**"TOE TOUCH"
:30 TV**

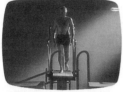

AVO: If you think people over 50 are still perfectly capable

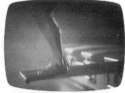

of touching their toes...

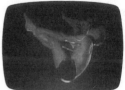

(PAUSE)

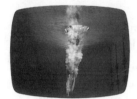

join the club.

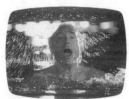

The Clarkson Health and Wellness Club.

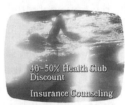

A free membership club that helps people over 50 lead healthy life-styles. With a health club discount,

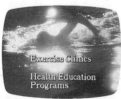

exercise clinics, health education programs and a lot more.

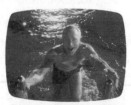

Plus extra privileges for those 65 and over.

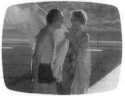

Find out more about the Clarkson Health and Wellness Club.

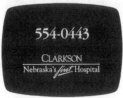

Call Clarkson Hospital. Once again, first in Nebraska.

Consider, for example, Children's Hospital in Columbus, Ohio, positioning itself as the provider of chemical dependency for adolescent services. It placed this ad, aimed at parents, in the daily paper. (See Exhibit 4-6.)

It placed another ad, aimed at students and peers who could bring pressure to bear on friends with addiction problems, in a range of high school newspapers, creative media planning, if difficult to find who to pay for the placements.

The public relations professionals took the campaign to another magnitude of exposure. Their "big idea": the hospital sponsored, with the main Columbus daily paper, a press conference on teen chemical dependency and how to help—*for high school journalists*. As a result, not only did the press conference and program receive extensive coverage from the daily paper, the story was picked up by other media; and most importantly, all those high school newspaper editors and reporters went back to their schools enlightened and energized to bring the story to where it would do the most good. Dozens of feature stories appeared in high school newspapers all over the state.

POSITIONING: SPECIAL QUESTIONS

Should the Hospital or the "Healthcare System" Be the Focus of Identity Development and Positioning?

(See Chapter 2, "Marketing an Integrated Healthcare Delivery System: The Fundamental Things Apply," for a more in-depth treatment of this question.)

Increasingly, it will be the "healthcare system" that will need to be positioned in the mind of the marketplace, not the hospital. "Healthcare system," in this context, does not refer to a "multihospital system," but to an integrated healthcare delivery system comprised of one or more hospitals, physicians, skilled nursing facilities, home care, and the other appropriate healthcare delivery sites.

Until now, brand equity has been deposited in the *hospital* by the marketplace. That was disturbing to executives and boards of multi-hospital systems. Numerous attempts were made to make the names of hospital systems "household words"—all to no avail. No one in the

RYNNE
Marketing Group

Our intervention program helps keep teenage alcohol and drug abuse where they belor

In school.

Many of the teenagers who seek help for an alcohol and drug problem shouldn't have to be taken out of school and away from home to deal with their problem.

That's why at Children's Hospital Guidance Centers, we've developed a brand new alcohol and drug intervention program that treats adolescents after school on an outpatient basis. This innovative program allows a teenager to remain in school and live at home while learning to cope with the stress of adolescence. Without the help of alcohol and drugs.

Outpatient vs. Inpatient Programs.

It has been shown that outpatient programs can be every bit as effective in helping many teenagers deal with alcohol or drug abuse as hospitalization. But without the disruption, the loss of schooling, and the stigma of isolation.

Find out more about our new ideas on teenage alcohol and drug intervention, including our outpatient Assessment and Continuing Care Programs. Call us confidentially at 431-7255.

Or check the box below for the times and topics in our free weekly Alcohol & Drug Education series held at our facilities: 740 Lakeview Plaza Blvd., Suite D, in Worthington.

Who knows more about your kid's health than Children's?

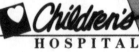

Children's
HOSPITAL

An Adolescent Health Service of Children's Hospital, Inc.

RYNNE
Marketing Group

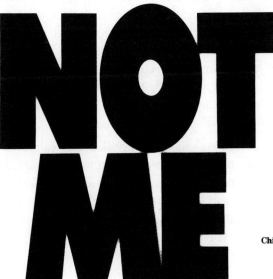

Four out of five Columbus area students would be right if they said this ad was not meant for them. The fifth would not.

This ad is about seeking help for an alcohol and drug problem.

At Children's Hospital Guidance Centers we offer an after school outpatient program that allows you to stay in school, live at home, and at the same time learn how to cope with the ups and downs of adolescence. Without alcohol and drugs.

If you or a friend are having a hard time saying no to alcohol or drugs, please say yes to help. And that way, when someone offers you a beer or a joint, you can say "not me".

Alcohol and Drug Services
Children's Hospital Guidance Centers
740-D Lakeview Plaza Blvd., Worthington

Phone 431-7255
(All Calls Confidential)

marketplace really cared—except in a peripheral way—whether or not his/her local hospital was part of a hospital system. People could understand issues such as enhanced purchasing power, corporate services, career ladders for executives, and enhanced access to capital when and if they were brought to their attention, but none of those features of a multihospital system really mattered to them in a central way. They were not the important issues when it came to their own purchase decisions. What they cared about was whether their local hospital was a good one or not.

Attempts to make the multihospital system the focus of attention for the general consumer were in many cases ego stroking for the leaders of the multihospital systems. There was little marketplace basis for the attempt—except in situations where the system was trying to establish multiple locations to support a managed-care strategy. The consumer, along with the physician, purchased the hospital, never a multihospital system. When ads appeared saying "Our multihospital system family cares for your family," the marketplace's reaction, when the ads were even noticed, was "say, what?"

All that however is about to change. Why? Because healthcare delivery and reimbursement are entering an era of profound change. Simply put, in the near future the consumer will be consciously choosing and purchasing one "integrated healthcare delivery system" instead of another. The object and content of the healthcare purchase decision will be "integrated healthcare delivery system" (although those words won't be used to describe the entity) and not the hospital.

That, of course, represents a very tall communications/education order. The marketplace will never understand a concept like "integrated healthcare delivery system" unless it has a very strong need to understand it. Eventually, the marketplace found it important enough to almost understand the concept of an HMO—at least enough to be able to accept or reject it as a purchase option. For the public to understand an even more complicated concept like "integrated healthcare delivery system" will take a correspondingly greater and pressing need to know. What is surprising is that that need to know is emerging. As the environment changes in ways that necessitate the development of the reality, so also the same changing environment is producing a climate where consumers will want to be able to understand what the reality is. What are those changes?

The ordinary working person and retiree will have a sharply felt, personal concern about the cost of healthcare because it will more and more directly effect his/her pocketbook.

Employees themselves will have to pick up the tab if they choose health coverage beyond the basic package or go outside the network of providers designated by the basic plan. As a result, when employees are selecting healthcare coverage they will be adding price to their traditional concerns of quality and convenience.

In that context they will have a need to know about an "integrated healthcare delivery system" because the integrated healthcare delivery system is the answer to the apparently contradictory desires for higher quality healthcare at a lower price. The response that the integrated healthcare delivery system makes is that there are great unnecessary costs in the way healthcare is currently delivered.

Those unnecessary costs can be taken out of the system if:

1) Hospitals and doctors work as one to rid patient care of unnecessary costs and steps. For example:

Because the ophthalmologists on staff at one hospital agreed that the hospital would purchase and stock two lenses—which the ophthalmologists agreed were the best lenses for most situations—instead of 12 different lenses, the hospital saved $500,000 per year through volume purchasing and more focused vendor negotiations.

Because the orthopedic surgeons at one hospital looked at the ways they were handling hip replacement cases—the great variety of their clinical approaches, use of tests, orders to nurses, timing of rehab's involvement, stocking of prostheses, approaches to incisions and sutures, etc.—they developed common protocols that led not only to better outcomes, but also to a shorter length of stay and reduced use of unnecessary resources. Annual savings: $2 million.

Cutting the costs of hospital care until recently was thought to be only a hospital management challenge. Cutting costs meant reducing staff and taking the fat out of the hospital budget. In most settings, those cuts have been made. There isn't more fat in the budget. More cuts will lead to lower quality patient care.

However, that is not where the big savings are to be had. The really huge reductions in costs of hospital care will come from a review of **medical resource decisions**—the decisions doctors make. Those savings can't be accomplished by hospital administrators. They can be realized only by doctors and hospital staff working together. The term "critical path analysis" describes the process physicians and hospital staff use to identify wasteful uses of resources that don't produce improved quality of care.

As the marketplace comes to understand how hospitals and doctors can, working together, reduce healthcare costs without short-changing quality, the marketplace will understand the first attribute of an integrated healthcare delivery system: doctors and hospitals working as one with common purposes and self interests.

2) Specialists will be used only if a primary-care physician indicates that it is medically necessary.

Currently, the populace often goes to specialists directly and often when it isn't necessary. Specialists are expensive. The second element of an integrated healthcare delivery system is that the primary-care physician services as gatekeeper to specialists.

3) Hospitals, as the most expensive part of the healthcare system, will be supplemented by services that provide patients appropriate care in less-expensive settings: step-down units, skilled nursing, facilities, day care, home care, and hospice and outpatient settings.

4) Transitions of patients between physicians and care settings are coordinated so there are no delays or wasted steps—improving quality, shortening recovery time, and lowering costs. This is the **case management** feature of an integrated healthcare delivery system.

5) Providers of care will be paid a given amount to take care of a person for the year.

It is in the providers' best interests, therefore, to either keep the patient healthy or provide care as efficiently and successfully (recurrence of illness means more costs to the provider) as possible. This is the capitated payment feature of an integrated healthcare delivery system.

In sum, working people who are looking for quality care at a price that won't mean paying a lot out of their own pockets, will begin to understand the concept of an integrated healthcare delivery system as the answer to their need for lower priced health care without cut-rate quality.

Currently, the employee chooses one insurance option over another. In the future, the content of the purchase decision will not be what it is now—namely, the choice first of a physician and the separate choice of a hospital based on the lists the insurance options offer. The content of the purchase decision will be the choice of one competing delivery system with one set of primary-care physicians/specialists/hospitals/nursing facilities/home care, etc., providing case management, critical path analysis, and prevention services for a fixed fee—and another set.

The future will belong to those who not only put together such systems most effectively, but also communicate most effectively how their systems are providing care at an efficient price without cutting quality.

A benefits manager at a major steel corporation articulated and exemplified the way many employees will be thinking in the future. He explained why he was so impressed with the presentation that Borgess Medical Center in Kalamazoo, Michigan, gave to his management team concerning its package price for open heart surgery. The price was so low in comparison to other open heart programs in the region that the hospital could pay for the transportation and lodging of the patient's whole family, make a profit, and still be lower than competitors. The benefits manager said:

> Borgess Medical Center showed us where they were a few years ago in terms of cost and quality, and where they are today, and how they got to where they are. They are working as a team with the physicians, nurses, etc. They had reduced length of stay. They've taken costs out of lab and X-ray components. They have measured and can demonstrate improvements in morbidity and mortality rates. The package they are offering includes the whole service from physicians to follow-up care. It includes transportation and lodging. [We were] impressed with the philosophy, the commitment, the results, and the presentation.

In short, he understood how the price could be lower—they **took the unnecessary costs out of the system,** the costs that are the result of hospitals and doctors and hospital-based specialists such as anesthesiologists, radiologists, and pathologists *not working together.* He saw that costs could be lower, without any loss of quality, in fact, with improved quality, if the providers had an incentive to work as one.

The pace of these trends will, of course, quicken if the government adopts a managed competition approach which will mandate healthcare delivery systems competing with one another at a fixed per capita fee. In this scenario, the reputation of one "provider set" (i.e., integrated healthcare delivery system) over another "provider set" will be the marketing key to success. The first "provider set" with the strongest reputation for the quality/price combination will have a distinct edge in the market, much as the hospital with the strongest reputation for quality had the edge in the old paradigm—when price hardly entered the consumer's mind as a decision variable.

It follows that in the new paradigm, it will be the "provider set" or "integrated healthcare delivery system" that should be the focus of positioning and brand-equity strategies. The name that will need to be the household word will be the name of the entire thing, not just the hospital. In this regard, there are some examples of hospitals that have already evolved in terms of brand equity into something more.

When people in Detroit, for example, say "Henry Ford" today they are not referring any longer to just Henry Ford Hospital. For the past 10 years, Henry Ford has been building ambulatory care satellites all around the metropolitan area, growing a PPO and HMO, adding hospitals, other healthcare settings, services, and physician groups to its system. It has placed the Henry Ford name on all its facilities and enterprises. As a result, the name "Henry Ford" now refers not just to the hospital but to the "whole thing."

The next step for a system like Henry Ford—now that it has evolved into a "whole thing," and its name embraces and points to a whole range of recognized facilities, services, and physicians, in addition to the main frame hospital—is to fill in for the market what benefit to them the system will be. Henry Ford has half the battle won. It is already perceived as much more than the sum total of its hospitals' brand equity. Most other systems across the country have very little name recognition.

Moreover, Henry Ford has already integrated most of its physicians into the organization. Many other hospitals and systems are still putting their Physician Hospital Organizations in place.

The transition from the old paradigm to the new will, however, never be total—even if the way healthcare is financed is totally revamped. The reputation of the mainframe hospital component of the integrated healthcare delivery system will still be important for the successful marketing of the system.

The reputation of a really fine hospital will still put a halo around the whole system of which it is a part. That is why the short-term strategy of some leading hospitals is explicitly a two-step strategy. For the next number of months, the strategy is to build and enhance the reputation of the hospital—both to enhance its appeal and draw additional business while the old paradigm still reigns, and to strengthen its halo effect for the system in the new paradigm. Then within X number of months, the strategy will change and total attention will be given to building the identity of the system.

In a Managed-Care Environment, Isn't Positioning to the General Public Irrelevant?

Some may argue that in a managed-care environment, marketing directly to the public doesn't make sense. The consumers in the general public aren't the key decision makers anymore, the managed-care companies and the employers are. It doesn't do any good for a hospital to market directly to the public if those very consumers are being directed away from the hospital because of their insurance coverage. All the marketing in the world won't bring them to a particular hospital if they are shut out of using that facility and directed elsewhere by their HMO or PPO. Save resources. Forget about positioning the hospital to the public. Invest those resources into managed care and employer contracting.

Response: In a managed-care environment, it's more important than ever to manage one's image in the mind of the consumer—because the stakes are higher than ever and because that's where the final purchase decision is being made.

It is true that the purchase decision is now often a three-step purchase decision in contrast to the days when it was only a two-step process. In the past, the marketing challenge for a hospital involved two customers: the physician and the consumer. The hospital wooed physicians to use it as their workshop and wooed the consumer to use its physicians, and when they had a direct choice for such services as emergency services or chemical dependency, to use the hospital directly.

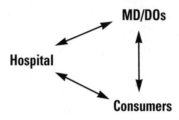

An effective marketer in this era could get a number of push/pull dynamics going to generate more business for the hospital.

1) Have the hospital so well perceived that consumers want to come to it, and base their choice of a physician on hospital affiliation. These consumers are "pulled" to the hospital and, consequently, to physicians through the power of reputation.

The hospital then "gives" that patient to one of its physicians, or the specialists at the hospital treat the patient and then "give" them to a primary-care physician.

2) Have the hospital so well perceived that consumers tell their physicians to admit them to the consumers' preferred hospital instead of to other hospitals in the market. This is another version of the "pull" strategy, but in this case, the consumer already has a physician. When the consumer is admitted, it might look like the physician is the decision maker, but actually, behind the physician is a very influential consumer.

3) Because of the excellent reputation of the hospital with the general public, physicians find the halo effect of practicing at that hospital helps them attract business. Physicians find it in their best interest, therefore, to direct patients to that hospital. In this case, hospital reputation "pulls" patients to the physicians and the physicians "push" patients to the hospital (pull and push combined).

4) The physicians find the hospital so satisfying a place to practice for themselves and their patients that they direct patients to use it instead of other choices. This is a purely "push" dynamic.

5) Physicians leave the choice of the hospital up to the patient and the patient chooses the hospital—because of its reputation (push *and* pull combination).

A savvy marketing-oriented hospital worked all five of these dynamics to its advantage. Even so, the conventional wisdom was: "Why waste resources marketing to the general public? The physician admits the patient. No patient is admitted or receives outpatient care at your hospital unless a physician signs the order. Save your resources. Invest in marketing to the physician." The response: There are many more opportunities for generating additional business than just strategy #4. Work all of them, not just one.

In a similar way, those who say, "In a managed-care environment there is no choice left," haven't really traced how the purchase decisions are made.

After the contracts between the healthcare providers and the managed-care entities have been signed, the job of marketing has only just begun. First, the employers have to be reached so that they will place this particular managed-care/healthcare provider option in front of their employees. Secondly, once the option is placed in front of the employees, the employees need to be reached and convinced that they should choose this particular option over others.

Trace the decision-making process for the various segments in a typical employee population. To keep it simple, take a situation in which the employer presents two competing plans: one with one insurer and set of providers, and another plan with a different insurer and provider set.

#1 The largest segment of employees reads down the list of physicians in each option to see if their personal physician is listed. The first cut of decision making: choose the option that causes the least disruption in one's personal life. Go with the status quo. Choose the option that allows one to stay with one's personal or family physician.

For this segment, the hospitals on the list are not as important a consideration as the physicians—either because the individuals in the segment are not looking beyond the choice of the physician to a possible hospitalization, or because they see the hospitals as undifferentiated, or because they trust that where their doctors practice will turn out fine for them.

From the standpoint of an individual hospital, the marketing strategy relating to this segment is to have as many primary-care physicians as possible who are preferred by these employees associated with the hospital. A secondary strategy is to work with those physicians to keep these employees well satisfied, stimulate word-of-mouth among them, and make sure they understand the consequences of their insurance choices.

For this segment, hospital image enhancement strategies to the general public are important only in a supportive way. It is important that the hospital not be negatively perceived by employees in a way that might drive the employee to look for other physicians. More positively, the reputation of the hospital should support the employees' choice of the physician.

#2 There are segments, however, for whom the hospital is a more important issue. For them, the hospital's reputation will more strongly enter their decision making process.

- Some have particular healthcare needs or conditions that make the hospital issue more important than to the typical consumer. For example, a woman who anticipates having a baby in the near future will scrutinize the list of hospitals to see if there are hospitals where she would like to deliver. A person with a heart condition will pay attention to the reputations of the hospitals for heart care, and so on. These employees will be open to changing their physician choice to access a particular hospital.

- Some employees don't have a personal physician.

- Some employees are dissatisfied with their personal physicians and are open to or looking for another.

- Some won't see their personal physicians on either list. As they consider the choice of a new physician, the reputation of the hospital where the physician practices enters in.

- For another segment, the reputation of the hospital is an overriding consideration, either because one hospital in the market is so well-perceived that the thought of being directed to other inferior hospitals is enough to make them change their physician choice or because they typically choose the hospital first and then their physician.

All these segments can be directly influenced in their managed-care choices by hospital positioning or image enhancement strategies.

Every year, employees choose anew their insurance/healthcare provider package.

Every year, there are opportunities for the hospital that understands where and how decisions are being made in a managed-care environment to influence those choices.

CHAPTER 5
Healthcare Marketing Plans That Get Results: A Proven Method

INTRODUCTION

Over the years, having developed marketing plans for many different healthcare lines of business—from HMO marketing plans to multi-specialty group practice marketing plans to cardiac, cancer, obstetrics, neurosciences, emergency department, orthopedic, and gastroenterology services marketing plans—in hundreds of healthcare organizations across the country, it is clear that there are important elements of *process* and *format* that raise the odds that a marketing plan will generate results.

Those time-tested discoveries and refinements are explained in this chapter.

The healthcare marketing executive pays attention to the *process* and the *format* for developing a marketing plan.

It is almost as important for the healthcare marketing executive to design a good process as it is to provide an effective format, because the healthcare marketing executive actually faces a double challenge. Not only should a well-implemented marketing plan produce results in the marketplace, it should also produce changes in consciousness internally. Producing a marketing plan that secures results is as much a political challenge as it is a technical one. Healthcare marketing executives don't lament this double challenge; they embrace it. Not only do they need to figure out the market and develop effective strategies to influence the market, they also need to figure out their colleagues and how to influence and motivate them. The energy and focus for implementing an effective marketing plan will be in direct proportion to the enthusiasm with which line managers and physicians embrace the marketing plan. Because the product and place "P"s—the way the services are designed and delivered—are the heart and soul of effective marketing, the amount of impact the marketing plan will have in the marketplace will be in direct proportion to the amount of elan generated within those responsible for carrying it out.

Before presenting the process and a format for constructing marketing plans that produce results, it is important first to be clear on what a marketing plan is and what it is not. There is frequently confusion within healthcare organizations concerning the difference between a marketing plan and a strategic plan, between a marketing plan and a business plan, and finally between a marketing plan and a marketing communications or promotion plan.

What a Marketing Plan Is Not

A Marketing Plan Is Not a Strategic Plan

The marketing plan is not a strategic plan. It differs from the strategic plan in five main ways. These differences are described below and illustrated in Figure 5-1.

1) purpose

2) time frame

3) degree of specificity

4) degree of line management and physician involvement in its development

5) orientation

A marketing plan is similar to a strategic plan in that neither type of plan is developed in a vacuum. They are designed to win a competitive game and are developed with an eye on what competitors are planning and how they will react. An attempt is made in both plans to be two moves ahead of the competitors. While similar in their strategic orientation, the **purposes** of the two plans are quite different.

The strategic plan focuses on "what businesses the organization should be in" while the marketing plan focuses on "bringing in the business." The strategic plan outlines what markets and services the organization should be entering, concentrating on, and/or de-emphasizing, whereas the marketing plan concentrates on making sure the markets the organization enters enter the organization, and the services that the organization concentrates upon end up being concentrated at the organization. The strategic plan sketches the broader strokes of what should be done and the marketing plan fills in how to get what should be done, done.

Second, the **time horizons** of the strategic plan and the marketing plan differ. The strategic plan arches over a three-to-five year time frame. More typically these days, because of the volatile environment, strategic plans are three years in duration and updated perhaps every other year. When organizations update their three year plans every year, it is hard to avoid the feeling of a paper chase.

The time frame of the marketing plan is *one* year—the coming fiscal year—and it is updated every year. Results are expected from a marketing plan within a shorter time frame.

The third difference between the two plans is the **degree of specificity** of the outcomes expected and the tactics to be implemented. The strategic plan states outcomes designed in terms of *goals*, which are measurable in *general* terms—e.g., to be a Center of Cancer Care Excellence by the year 199– or to be the leading Center for Cancer Care by 199–. The outcomes articulated in a strategic marketing plan are not goal statements but *objectives*, which are clearly and *specifically measurable*—e.g., to increase the number of radiation therapy patients cared for by our hospital from X to Y by the end of the year, or to be rated the number one cancer treatment center in the area by 90 percent of the area general surgeons and internists, or to increase the number of direct contracts with area employers from X to Y.

The fourth difference between the strategic plan and the marketing plan is the **degree of involvement** required of physicians and line managers in their development. The development of a good strategic plan requires input from, understanding of, and support for the plan by physicians and line managers. The development of the marketing plan not only requires physician and line manager input, understanding, and support, it requires their intimate involvement and ownership. It requires ownership by those responsible for the product and place "P"s, namely the physicians and line managers. It is enough for a plan that describes "what businesses the organization should be in" to have the general understanding and support of its key constituents. A plan that specifies "how the organization will bring in the business" has to be more than a plan that physicians endorse, it has to be a plan that they own.

The final difference between a strategic plan and a marketing plan is in their **orientations**.

A strategic plan is investment oriented. A marketing plan is revenue oriented. The key question asked in the strategic plan is: How do we take our limited resources and invest them in such a way as to have a long-term, profitable future? This investment orientation at times makes internal constituents wary of strategic planning because if one service or sector of an organization receives an infusion of resources, that means, in a zero sum game, that someone else will not be receiving those resources. A marketing plan, on the other hand, is not part of a zero sum game. A good marketing plan should produce more resources for all. As a marketing plan generates additional business and additional revenue, or in the new era, less use of resources due to behavior change, the organization has a stronger bottom line. That means there will be more for everyone. That usually means that internal constituents approach marketing expectantly, not warily.

Figure 5-1: Differences Between a Strategic Plan and a Marketing Plan

	Strategic Plan	Marketing Plan
Content	What businesses the organization should be in	How to bring in the business
Time Frame	3 to 5 years	1 year
Degree of Specificity	**Goals**, measurable in **general** terms	**Objectives,** measurable in **specific** terms
Level of MD and Line Manager Involvement in Development	Input, understanding, and support	Input, understanding, support, ownership, and commitment
Orientation	Investment oriented	Revenue oriented

A Marketing Plan Is Not a Business Plan

A marketing plan is part of a business plan.

A business plan presented for a business funding decision will have a number of components beyond the marketing strategy section. It will include a description of the product and sponsoring organization; the track record of those requesting the investment; the organizational structure; an outline of anticipated obstacles to success; and a competitive assessment and a financial plan including capitalization, operating statement, cash flow analysis, and an anticipated return on investment schedule. While the marketing feasibility and strategy sections are the bedrock of a solid business plan, they are only parts of the whole.

A Marketing Plan Is Not a Marketing Communications or Promotion Plan

The promotion plan is part of the marketing plan.

The marketing plan will include a promotion plan, an important section that outlines how to best reach the target segments for a particular service, how to best allocate resources across a given schedule of communication methods, and the appropriate content and the tone for each element of the campaign.

But as important as the promotion plan is, a marketing plan will include much more. It will provide the information profile that shapes the decisions in the communications plan, and it will give primacy to the product and place "P"s of the marketing mix. Recognizing that the worst thing to do with a bad product is promote it, and that most of the time in healthcare the reason why a given service is not living up to expectations is not the lack of promotion as much as it is the lack of a customer-satisfying service, the marketing plan takes all deliberate care that the service itself and the way it is delivered are up to par to the customers' evaluative criteria. If, for example, the reason why people are staying away from an emergency room is the perceived lack of physician quality or wait times are out of line, the marketing plan will give priority to addressing these issues before it invests in promotion.

What Is a Marketing Plan?

A marketing plan is the document developed before the annual budget cycle that describes the priority objectives the organization will achieve through marketing in a given year, how it will achieve them, who is responsible for carrying them out, in what sequence, with what resources, and with what return.

Consequently, the formats for developing a strategic plan and a marketing plan will be quite different. Even their use of information will have a different slant and spin.

THE PROCESS AND FORMAT FOR DEVELOPING A HEALTHCARE MARKETING PLAN

The **process** of developing an effective marketing plan in a healthcare organization will have four characteristics, and the **format** for developing an effective marketing plan will also have four characteristics.

First, the **process** for developing a marketing plan will have the following features:

1) The process doesn't end up having some people feel stuck with responsibilities for things that they can't really influence or accomplish.

2) The process makes marketing a practical, decision-making exercise, not a theoretical or political exercise.

3) The process asks for just the right amount of commitment and time from those involved in developing it.

4) The process links marketing planning with the other important management systems within a healthcare organization, in particular the budgeting and evaluation systems.

Secondly, the **format** for developing effective healthcare marketing plans will have the following features:

1) It will grow out of a rich review of relevant marketing information.

2) It will begin with measurable marketing objectives and end with stating the worth of the objectives if achieved.

3) It will utilize a simple, easy-to-use process transferable to other situations but incorporating all the best of classic marketing.

4) It will produce a steady stream of insights and discoveries for participants as they follow the format.

The Process of Producing Effective Healthcare Marketing Plans

The Process of Producing a Marketing Plan Doesn't End Up with Some People Feeling Stuck with Responsibilities for Things That They Can't Really Influence or Accomplish.

To produce a healthcare marketing plan that gets results, it is important to involve all the key actors involved in the design and delivery of a service, so that they are not caught by surprise after the fact by someone else's marketing plan that has implications for them, and so that they can understand and fully embrace the strategies and tactics in the marketing plan. Therefore, it is important to name a marketing "team" to develop a marketing plan.

For example, a marketing team developing a marketing plan for an emergency department will need to involve a number of key actors important for effectively designing emergency services. The team will be comprised of emergency department physician leadership, nursing leadership, registration and billing leadership, as well as marketing staff members. Moreover, if the strategies and tactics for strengthening an emergency department are likely to need the participation and support of the departments of radiology and pathology, leadership from those departments are involved on the front end as well. To provide a quality emergency service in a timely fashion will involve the active collaboration of a number of departments and functions within a medical center.

Involving leadership from these different disciplines and departments also means that changes that need to take place in those departments and functions will be assigned to leadership from those departments and functions. The responsibility for implementing the marketing plan, therefore, won't fall to people who don't feel they can influence behavior in related disciplines. If, for example, changes in physician practice style, behavior, or scheduling are required in order to grow the business of an emergency department, it is important that the physicians take responsibility for those initiatives. If nursing is left with implementation responsibility all by itself, it ends up feeling powerless and frozen in place.

A marketing team, moreover, should have different levels of responsibility assigned to it from the beginning. It makes sense for a vice-president-level person to serve as the lead for the development of a marketing plan and its implementation. This saves unnecessary organizational stress and duress on department managers. Achievement of a major healthcare marketing objective requires the active collaboration of multiple actors. Coordination of all the actors requires as senior a person as possible. A department manager typically does not enjoy the authority to secure cooperation from other sectors of the organization. If they succeed, it is on the strength of their natural leadership and persuasion abilities.

A vice-president, on the other hand, or a senior line executive, is in a peer relationship to other vice-presidents to whom other departments report. Placing lead responsibility with a member of the senior management team makes achievement less dependent on personal charisma—which may be in short supply—and more on position power, which is built in. In a healthy organization, cooperation between peers within senior management secures cooperation from their departments with one another.

The Process of Producing the Marketing Plan Makes Marketing a Practical Decision-Making Exercise, Not a Theoretical or Political Exercise.

A marketing team's mandate is very different from a "task force-run-amok's" mandate. A marketing team is focused on solving a problem, namely how to strengthen and/or grow a particular business line. That makes the marketing planning exercise eminently practical, not theoretical.

One major medical center, for example, once convened a task force to consider the future of its cancer care services. Their mandate: envision an ideal cancer care service. The task force, comprised of cancer care professionals of various persuasions all concerned with protecting their respective turfs, had been meeting for well over a year and had not yet agreed on the definition of cancer care services. All too often in healthcare, task forces are asked to develop position papers and complete, what is in effect, a theoretical task. Clinical professionals typically are not that skilled at philosophizing. They are, however, superb problem solvers. A practical setting fits them much more suitably than a theoretical, philosophizing setting. When the mandate of the task force was changed to the practical marketing challenge, namely "how do we grow our cancer care services," the content and the tone of the sessions changed immediately. All participants were able to get down to business.

Neither is a marketing planning process a political bartering session. A typical strategic planning task force begins with the premise that resources are limited and only certain areas will be receiving an infusion of capital. As a result, strategic planning can be highly volatile and political. If a limited pie is to be divvied up, many begin politicking for their shares. A marketing planning process, on the other hand, focuses on enlarging the pie available. It begins with a practical challenge: how do we grow this business effectively and efficiently? Turf protection is subsumed into turf enlargement.

The entire process of developing a marketing plan is conducted in a problem-solving mode. Position papers aren't presented for participants to pick apart and critique. Instead, options are laid out and selected. Participants are tapped for their insights and suggestions. Nominal group techniques are used to make sure all get to have their say, not just those who are dominant personalities, inveterate talkers, or in prestige positions. The process itself contributes to building the team—all focused on action, not discussion, results not plans, gains not posturing.

The Process of Developing a Marketing Plan Asks Just the Right Amount of Time and Commitment from Participants.

Healthcare managers and physicians who carry a management responsibilities within healthcare have so many demands on their time and talents, it is very important to avoid the feeling that they are being asked to do "one more thing." It's very important, therefore, to spell out just what the commitment is and how it will fit into the rest of their responsibilities. The following schedule is recommended to prevent some of those misgivings and shying away from involvement. The schedule proceeds in three basic steps, each requiring no more than two hours involvement from participants. It requires a total of six hours of their time. This schedule tells them what will be done, how it will be done, and who will be doing it. It limits to a manageable amount of time their involvement and is scheduled around the rhythm of the rest of their responsibilities. It proceeds in three marketing planning modules.

At the first session (two-hours long) marketing team members will:

- Review the relevant marketing information. Conduct a SWOT analysis (strengths, weaknesses, opportunities, and threats analysis);
- Set provisional marketing objectives;
- Select the priority market segments for the marketing plan; and
- Begin brainstorming on effective strategies and tactics.

The marketing staff and other support people will, before the first session, put together the marketing information that will help shape the development of the marketing plan. They are doing the staff or leg work for the line managers and physicians. Between the first and the second sessions, the marketing staff will put together the results of the first session and draft, in effect, a first go at the marketing strategies and tactics.

At the second session (two hours long) marketing team members will:

- Review draft strategies and tactics;
- Begin to prioritize the strategies and tactics; and
- Begin to assign responsibilities.

At the third session (two hours long) marketing team members will:

- Complete the assignment of responsibilities, timing, and resources;
- Establish the worth of the marketing objectives if achieved; and
- Review and refine a marketing communications plan designed to reach both internal and external audiences.

This schedule has the merit of fully involving the marketing team participants. It is not just a top-of-mind, shallow involvement. Marketing team members are fully engaged through this schedule in thinking through the important issues of effective marketing. On the other hand, it is not an onerous obligation. They are not meeting forever. It is a very efficient, productive use of their time and talents.

The Process of Constructing a Marketing Plan for Results Links Marketing Planning with the Other Important Management Systems Within a Healthcare Organization.

The budgeting and evaluation systems are particularly important. The development of key marketing plans in a healthcare organization should, on an annual basis, precede the development of the budget. In this way, strategy will dictate resources rather than the other way around.

This means that the marketing plans that promise the greatest return on investment are likely to receive the most resources for achieving those objectives. Linking marketing plans with the budget begins to build in an "ROI" attitude towards marketing and confidence in marketing's ability to contribute. Good marketing produces substantial financial returns within a stated amount of time. It is not just the promotion part of marketing, however, that produces results; it is the orchestration of the entire marketing mix that brings those results. It's the marketing plan, not the communications plan alone, that produces those results. Such an attitude reinforces the priority of the product and placement "P"s of the marketing mix and does not put unnecessary expectations on marketing communications for generating business.

In turn, the link with the budget reemphasizes the importance of measurable, achievable marketing objectives and aggressive, well-coordinated implementation of the strategies to achieve those objectives. This in turn sets up a straightforward rhythm of evaluation of marketing's contribution to the organization.

If senior management has selected the appropriate marketing priorities and the marketing teams develop effective marketing plans, and then carry through on the tactics that promise results, the organization should be able to review those results in a steady, measured way. The process of producing a marketing plan that gets results begins and ends with an expectation that the results will be watched and measured. "It's not what you expect, it's what you inspect" that produces results.

The Format for Developing Healthcare Marketing Plans That Get Results

Hallmark #1: A marketing plan that generates results begins with and grows out of a rich review of relevant marketing information.

Good marketing planning, like good strategic planning, begins with well analyzed, good information. The information, however, that the marketing executive finds most helpful and will labor to present to a marketing team has a different spin and content than the information presented for purposes of strategic planning. This is illustrated in Figure 5-2. Even the title of a report developed at the outset of a strategic planning exercise is different from the title of a report developed to launch a marketing planning process. The title of the data report for strategic planning is popularly entitled "an environmental assessment." The title of the data report that will launch a marketing planning exercise is better called a "market opportunity report."

Figure 5-2: The Planner and the Marketer: Different Approaches to Data

Environmental Assessment	Market Opportunity Report
To prepare for what's going to happen to you	To prepare for you to make it happen
Where to sow	Where to reap
Size of business that's out there	Size of business that can be shifted
Aware of what's coming	Aware of what's possible
Where the innovations are	Where the choices are

In an environmental assessment, information is gathered that will facilitate the decisions about "what businesses to be in and where to make successful investments." The information is designed to prepare an organization to meet its future. It points out areas where the organization should be investing or sowing its resources, and ranks, through portfolio analysis, a range of business investment priorities. The strategic plan is focused on identifying what is coming over the horizon in terms of environmental change and industry innovation.

A market opportunity report, on the other hand, is not as focused on where an organization should invest or sow its resources for future return, it is much more focused on identifying current opportunities for immediate return. A market opportunity report is very focused on opportunities that currently exist for growing existing business lines. It focuses on the amount of business that can be shifted in the marketplace, given current opportunities and certain strategic moves, as opposed to just describing the size of businesses that are currently out there and ready for investment. It emphasizes not just what is coming, but also what is possible. It focuses on where and how choices are being made, not just on what is happening.

An effective marketing planning process begins with a review of relevant marketing information. Included among the relevant marketing information, of course, is performance trend information concerning particular services and practitioners: market share analysis, profitability analysis, payor mix information, and demographic information as it relates to changing business potential.

These are all important pieces of information, but the following four analyses are especially valuable for identifying current **opportunities** in the marketplace. They serve as the core of a market opportunity report.

There are four categories of information that are particularly important for the market opportunity report.

1) Information and analysis on how business is currently coming through the door

2) "Gusher" information and analysis

3) 80/20 information

4) SWOT information

Source of business information and analysis

Many times in healthcare, leadership doesn't have a very clear understanding of how business is currently coming in the door. It is, therefore, typically the first order of business to "map" the sources of business. This doesn't refer to patient origin information. All patient origin information tells leadership is the geographic location of the customer's residence. At times, it is correlated with decision making by intermediary decision makers, but, of itself, it doesn't describe how business is coming through the door. To see that, it is important to trace the distinct contributors to the business in terms of distinct decision-making segments. See Figures 5-3 through 5-5.

A simple example appears in Figure 5-3 below: A Houston neurosurgery group's map of how business comes in the door.

Figure 5-3: Houston Neurosurgery Practice Map

| 20% Emergency Room | 15% Trauma |
| | 5% Self-Referral |

20% Physician Referral	5% Neurologist
	5% Orthopedic
	10% Primary Care (Family Practice, General Practitioner, Internal Medicine)

| 60% Self-Referral | 50% Family or Friend |
| | 10% General Reputation |

Note the implications of such a map. This, of course, is an atypical neurosurgery practice in that most of its business comes from word-of-mouth. Compare that to another neurosurgery practice in the State of Virginia.

Figure 5-4: Virginia Neurosurgery Practice Map

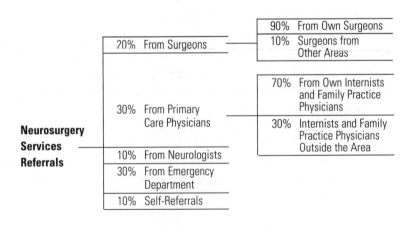

This map indicates a more typical neurosurgery practice.

In the Houston situation, the map points out the six basic ways to grow the business, given the three contributing streams—grow the *size* of each of the three streams collaboratively with those contributors. And then secondly, increase the *share* of business from those contributing streams—another three ways to grow the business.

This neurosurgery group (Figure 5-3) has two promising strategies open to it as revealed through the map. One, grow the word-of-mouth business even more aggressively. This practice had never actively nurtured its primary source of business, namely former patients, but patients sent them business anyway. Once patients completed treatment, the practice never communicated with the patients again. Former patients, however, were so satisfied that they frequently recommended this practice to friends and acquaintances they met who talked of similar back problems. The practice was mainly oriented to relieving back pain, and therefore able to generate substantial word-of-mouth or patient referral business.

Consequently, a successful tactic in the marketing plan was to keep in touch more consistently and aggressively with the large pool of former patients through a periodic personalized newsletter providing interesting information on the neurosurgeons and their practice as well as lay-oriented information on advancements in neurosurgery. This simple tactic prompted even more patients to refer word-of-mouth business to them.

The second strategy targeted a few of the primary-care physician practices in the market that weren't totally locked in to other providers of neurosurgical services. The practice initiated a targeted outreach effort to these specific primary-care physicians and generated additional business from them.

The neurosurgical group in Virginia, on the other hand (Figure 5-4), in reviewing its map of business, could see that it had additional opportunities "over the mountains" with referring physicians that they had not paid much attention to. Moreover, they could see that by changing their protocols and allowing patient referrals, there could be substantial additional business from that contributing source as well.

Mapping how business comes in the door does a number of important things for a marketing team. First, it roots them in reality. No more guesses or anecdotal information on how business comes to them. Second, it shows graphically the relative size of various key customer constituents and their dependence on those constituents. Third, it points out graphically where anomalies are and/or opportunities. Once anomalies have been surfaced, they can be addressed and fixed. Once opportunities have been surfaced, they can be taken advantage of. Fourth, it gets a marketing team to look at its business from the standpoint of the marketplace.

Take, for example, another simple map of how business comes in the door.

Figure 5-5: How the Business Comes in the Door

20% or 6,000	MD Referral	Convenience Reasons	70% or 4,200
		Referred for Emergency	30% or 1,800
40% or 12,000	Self Referral	Brought by Someone Else	50% or 6,000
		On One's Own	50% or 6,000
30% or 9,000	Ambulance Service	Private	60% or 5,400
		Public	40% or 3,600
10% or 3,000	Industrial Medicine	Contract	20% or 600
		Ad Hoc	80% or 2,400

In reviewing this map of how business comes in the door, the emergency physicians realized that they had never thought of the emergency department business in this way before. They didn't realize how much business was actually being sent to them through the word-of-mouth influence of paramedics and prehospital providers. They didn't realize how large the potential was for profitable business from the injured worker segment. They didn't realize how much of their business was actually chest pain related, and how much more of that business existed in the marketplace.

Uncovering such information concerning how business comes in the door can either be straightforward or very difficult. The more marketing oriented a healthcare organization is, the more likely it will be keeping and tracking such information. A side benefit that emerges from attempting to put together source of business information is the realization that a clinical service or entity within the healthcare organization needs to begin keeping such information. It is golden information for any business line that is trying to grow and shift market share.

"Gusher" information and analysis

The second type of information that is particularly useful for a marketing team is a "gusher" matrix. Whenever a marketing team is developing a marketing plan for a business line, it needs to first make some selections from within the business line of aspects or clinical services within the business line that are particularly promising. That selection requires the ability to see the leverage points for revenue generation in the short term and the ability to see how particular choices contribute to the overall competitive positioning of the business line in the longer term. A marketing team will, therefore, at the outset, select its "gushers," services with significant revenue potential in the short term. If the marketing team taps a particular gusher, it can be much more successful and profitable rather quickly. Such a selection requires facility with handling a number of evaluative criteria all at once.

When comparing services with one another to decide which ones deserve the most attention and focus from the marketing plan, a marketing team, in effect, uses the following criteria, which are explained below and illustrated in Figures 5-6 and 5-7.

- Profitability

    All things being equal, services which have potential to subsidize others will receive priority attention.

- Possesses significant clinical strength

    All things being equal, the service which already has excellent physician or clinical leadership will be a higher priority than the service which has promise but still requires recruitment. The service with strong clinical quality will perform better in the marketplace than the one which is still on the way.

- Competitive vulnerability

    Even if a service does not currently have market share, if competitors are vulnerable on some important score such as leadership, location, responsiveness, or quality—that might signal a gusher.

Figure 5-6: Ratings on Business Development Selection Criteria

Service	Clinical Strengths	Positioning Power	Profit	Competitor Vulnerability	Underserved Segments	Small Investment	Spin-Off Revenue	Product Champion	Total Score

Note: ● = Highly correlated (9 points) △ = Marginally correlated (1 point)
○ = Somewhat correlated (3 points) - = Not correlated (No points)

Figure 5-7: Business Development Plan for a Neuroscience Institute

Niche Services	Clinical Strength	Competitive Vulnerability	Income Potential	Managed Care Support & Interest	Investment Cost	Total
1. Balance Disorders	◉	◉	○	△	◉	31
2. Pediatric Neurosurgery	○	◉	◉	○	△	25
3. Diagnostic Testing						
• Sleep Disorders	◉	○	◉	○	○	27
• Intraoperative Monitoring	◉	◉	◉	△	◉	37
• EEG, Evoked Potentials	◉	◉	○	△	◉	31
• Transcranial Doppler	○	◉	△	△	○	17
4. Epilepsy Service	◉	○	◉	◉	○	33
5. Stroke Service (not yet ready)						
6. Spine Instrumentation	◉	○	◉	○	○	27
7. Neurosurgery	◉	△	◉	◉	○	31
• Radiosurgery	◉	○	◉	○	◉	33

Legend: ◉ = Strongly correlated (9 points)   △ = Minimally correlated (1 point)
○ = Correlated (3 points)   = No correlation (No points)

- Underserved segments in the marketplace

  If particular segments in a market are going overlooked or are undersatisfied, their allegiance can be changed or secured. Depending on the size of the segments and the degree of their dissatisfaction, this criterion may indicate a gusher.

- Amount of investment already made

  All things being equal, the service that has already received a significant investment of capital in terms of equipment, facility, or staff might deserve priority status over another that has not received such an investment in the past. Making it a priority in a given year might be just what is required to take it over the top and to start earning dividends on past investments.

- Amount of investment required

  The smaller the investment required and the greater the potential leverage of the investment, the more attractive is the service as a gusher.

- Degree of spin-off revenue

  Some services produce significantly greater indirect or referral revenue than others. Some services produce more long-term customers than others. While not gushers in terms of direct revenue, they may be gushers in terms of overall revenue or contribution to the business.

- Presence of a product champion

  All things being equal, when a service is led by someone who "makes things happen," that is a very important indicator of a gusher. Without a product champion, a service will probably not be effectively marketed because it lacks a rallying force and cohesive power who can bring all the component parts together and motivate the whole team to go after the marketplace. At times, some services, weak on other evaluative criteria, end up performing beyond expectations because of a strong product champion.

- Positioning power

  The second facility required of a management team in selecting a slate of priority marketing objectives is the ability to chart how the choice of high-profile marketing initiatives influences the organization's overall positioning. Recognizing that various services have more symbolic impact on the marketplace than others in terms of overall reputation for quality, service, and other dimensions of positioning strategy.

Some services have the cachet to spread a halo effect over the rest of a business line. The more closely related to saving lives a particular service is, the more it has halo power. That is why open heart surgery, neurosurgery, and trauma services have such positioning power for an organization as a whole. They convey an aura of serious life and death medicine. Similarly, within a business line, some services have more positioning power than others.

This gusher matrix should be completed by the marketing team in a group session. The marketing department should present information that is available that helps them make decisions concerning each of the boxes in the matrix, but the matrix is designed to bring forth different perspectives on the ratings, build consensus behind a final decision, and correct for prejudices within the team. Through the combination of objective data and subjective between-the-lines insights, the marketing team is able to make a determination concerning the choice of gushers.

The matrix is useful for a clinical service with many contributing sublines of business. More typically, that occurs in a teaching or university hospital setting. Completing such a matrix keeps the marketing team from making a bland, undifferentiated offering to the marketplace. In the matrix above, for example, instead of talking about neurosciences in general, the marketing plan is able to develop strategies behind the components of the service that will produce the greatest return. Marketing balance disorders and epilepsy services will be very different from the marketing of back pain services.

The matrix illustrated in Figure 5-8 is particularly useful for a senior management team selecting among alternatives for the organization's marketing slate.

80/20 Information

The third type of information to present to the marketing team at the outset of a marketing planning process is any relevant 80/20 percent information. Applying Pareto's law to the source of business information will frequently make more obvious significant opportunities that have been overlooked. The heavy user principal or Pareto's law states

Figure 5-8: Ratings on Business Development Selection Criteria

Service	Clinical Strengths	Positioning Power	Profit	Competitor Vulnerability	Underserved Segments	Small Investment	Spin-Off Revenue	Product Champion	Total Score
Oncology	●	●	○	○	○	●	○	●	48
Cardiovascular	●	●	○	◁	○	○	●	◁	38
Rehab	○	○	●	●	○	▪	○	◁	31
Obstetrics	●	●	○	●	○	●	○	◁	46
Mammography	○	◁	◁	●	●	◁	○	▪	27
Neurology	○	●	○	●	●	◁	●	●	52
Emergency Dept.	●	●	◁	○	◁	▪	●	●	41
Orthopedics	○	○	○	●	●	○	●	▪	39
Outpatient Surg.	●	◁	○	◁	▪	◁	◁	◁	17

Note:
● = Highly correlated (9 points)
○ = Somewhat correlated (3 points)
◁ = Marginally correlated (1 point)
▪ = Not correlated (No points)

that 20 percent of customers will provide 80 percent of the business and is frequently true in healthcare marketing.

Profiling that 20 percent gives insight into the marketplace. If more people in the marketplace fit the profile of the heavy user segment, there may be significant untapped opportunity.

A hospital in South Carolina, for example, was working on a marketing plan for recruiting additional physicians to its staff. It currently had 35 member physicians on its medical staff, and its growing population could support an additional 10. Most of them were in primary-care specialties. The hospital had been frustrated using physician recruitment firms and had decided to take responsibility for physician recruitment in-house.

In reviewing the past profile of recruitment efforts, it was asked if the previous 10 physicians that had come on staff within the last two years had anything in common. Was there a profile of success that could be drawn? At first, the members of the marketing team, which included a cross-section of physicians and the administrative team, thought there was nothing that these physicians had in common. One had come as a locum tenens and decided to stay. One had come because he experienced a "Ducks Unlimited" social event and was impressed by the community. Another came because of a friend. Upon further reflection, however, the marketing team realized that all 10 of the physicians had grown up within 30 miles of the hospital. They hadn't realized how strongly the 80/20 principal was at work.

Once they saw this profile, they devised some previously overlooked strategies and tactics. They had never invited any residents or medical students who had grown up in the area for a personal visit. They hadn't involved such soon to be physicians with any members of the medical staff. They had never wooed or targeted residents of the area who had decided to become physicians. The marketing plan outlined a number of very productive tactics including summertime occupations in physicians' offices for medical students, and an active holiday program dinner for nurturing relationships between leading medical staff members and residents who grew up in the region and were completing their programs at various residency programs across the country.

Another example—a hospital administrator in South Dakota was jubilant because he had finally recruited his one physician, which would allow the hospital to remain open. For two years, he had kept the hospital going through the efforts of locum tenens physicians. When asked what the key variable was in drawing the physician to his hospital, he responded, "It turned out to be clean air, clean water." He realized that his recruitment challenge would have been much more effective if he had used *Field and Stream* for his advertisements instead of *The New England Journal of Medicine*.

SWOT analysis information

The final type of information that is particularly valuable for effective marketing planning is SWOT analysis information: strengths, weaknesses, opportunities, and threats analysis that frequently produce immediate in-sights into priority tactics for a marketing plan.

When marketing team members identify the weaknesses of a business line, they are typically zeroing in immediately on important product and place issues in terms of the marketing mix. The flip side of weaknesses is typically opportunities.

It is hard, for example, for a marketing team that has articulated as one of the major weaknesses of the cardiac services program of a teaching hospital the fact that the marketplace sees this service as "resident run," to not address that issue in the marketing plan. Even though it is a very difficult and politically charged issue, it is important that attending physicians step in and begin to project a different reputation for the service and not allow residents to behave as they have behaved in the past. It is difficult for an emergency services marketing team, who indicate in the SWOT analysis that the triage function is not located appropriately, nor staffed adequately, and that it is the cause of much dissatisfaction among their customers, not to address the enhancement of the triage service as a key "product" element in the marketing plan.

In summary, effective marketing plans begin with a review of relevant marketing information which is more relevant to the degree that it points out current opportunities in the marketplace.

Out of the sea of possible data to be reviewed, the marketing staff selects the information that is the most relevant. Trend information will be relevant, but it will only describe the service as it has functioned and currently functions. More important is information that points to and dramatizes opportunities for the marketing team. Source of business information, 80/20 profiles, gusher matrices, and SWOT analyses are especially valuable for revealing hidden opportunities.

Hallmark #2: **A format should make sure that a marketing team sets relevant marketing objectives at the front end, and establishes the worth of the marketing objectives when the plan is completed.**

A format for developing marketing plans that get results makes very clear the importance of measurable, but appropriate, marketing objectives, because, in the long run, achieving those measurable objectives will be the surest way for resources to be committed to marketing the next time around.

The marketing team needs to understand the seriousness with which the organization will take the marketing objectives. These are not just wishes or vague intentions, they will be honest-to-goodness targets that leadership will be held accountable for securing. The achievement of promised marketing/business development objectives will be a key part of one's annual evaluation. Those that set timid marketing objectives will be perceived and evaluated as timid. Those that set unreal objectives will not be believed the next time. Those that set stretching, yet achievable, objectives and deliver on their promises will be rewarded and valued.

Selecting the appropriate measurable marketing objectives will take some education of marketing team members by the marketing professionals. A good place to start, as a primer, is with the ladder of marketing achievement illustrated in Figure 5-9.

Figure 5-9: The Ladder of Marketing Achievement

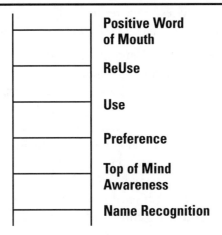

Positive Word of Mouth

ReUse

Use

Preference

Top of Mind Awareness

Name Recognition

Appropriate marketing objectives can be set anywhere along this ladder—under the old paradigm of healthcare decision making—depending on where the market currently stands vis-à-vis the organization.

It is appropriate to set **awareness** objectives such as "X percent increase in name recognition" when a service is newly established, or is going after the market in an aggressive way for the first time. A new managed-care offering may need to first gain name recognition in a given period before it can legitimately be expected to attract additional contracts. Moreover, name recognition objectives are quite appropriate when an organization is trying to establish a firm brand identity. More often, however, name recognition is not the appropriate focus for the marketing plan. A well-established healthcare marketing organization already has sufficient name recognition and needs to move the market up the marketing ladder.

It is not possible to jump over the rungs of the ladder. Name recognition precedes and serves as the foundation for the next rung of the ladder, namely top-of-mind recognition.

A legitimate objective for a marketing plan may be a top-of-mind awareness objective such as, "Our hospital will be the first hospital mentioned by the market when asked about sports medicine services. In this case, for example, top-of-mind awareness for sports medicine services is 28 percent, and the hospital wants to move from 28 percent to 40 percent of the market spontaneously thinking of us when they hear the term sports medicine." Top-of-mind awareness objectives are appropriate when a business line or a healthcare organization is trying to clearly differentiate itself from others. When it wants to be known for particular facets or services, it moves beyond mere name recognition to a differentiated position in the marketplace.

A name may be recognized and an organization may be thought of spontaneously for a particular attribute or service, but even more importantly, moving up the ladder of marketing achievement, is the market's **preference** for a particular organization. It is possible for an organization to be at the top of one's consciousness, but still not be preferred. Underlying the development of increased preference is a whole set of issues that enter into a judgment of preference. An organization's overall image and reputation enters into the market's intention to use the organization. Moreover, issues of access and geographic proximity and connection with a preferred caregiver are all involved in the preference rating. "To increase the percent of the market that prefers us for a particular service from X to Y" is more aggressive than mere name recognition or top-of-mind awareness. It works at establishing mind share with the marketplace. That is the next step to increased market share.

If a marketing team thinks that in a given time frame the market can be moved up the ladder from name recognition through top-of-mind awareness through preference to use, then utilization objectives are the appropriate marketing objectives. An objective such as "to increase market share from X to Y, or to increase the volume of elective surgeries from X to Y," is an appropriate and, of course, preferred objective to the mere "making a splash or managing image" outcomes lower down on the marketing ladder.

Recognizing that in a service business customer satisfaction becomes the root of ongoing success, both in terms of repeat business and word-of-mouth business, leads a marketing team to consider setting a readiness-to-recommend or readiness-to-return type objective. The marketing plan following from such an objective would put heavy emphasis on service excellence and solving issues that keep customers from being delighted.

Finally, the pinnacle of marketing achievement, especially in a service business, is to focus on word-of-mouth testimony objectives. An objective such as, "85 percent of our customers will rate us a 5 on a 1-to-5 scale" is much more challenging than setting a simple average customer satisfaction objective. By focusing on the delight end of the scale, the marketing plan can generate substantial additional business.

Setting Marketing Objectives Under the New Paradigm

The marketing ladder is quite appropriate in the old paradigm and between the times, and is even appropriate for certain segments of the marketplace before capitation has taken a strong hold in a given marketplace. But marketing objectives in a capitated setting take on a different content. There is a different ladder of marketing achievement for guiding the development of marketing objectives under the new paradigm. In a capitated setting, the first step on the marketing ladder is awareness of inappropriate and resource-wasting behaviors. Moreover, it is important for the market to be spontaneously aware of options to those kinds of behaviors, and finally, to not use certain expensive services and instead utilize less expensive and more appropriate options.

An emergency department marketing plan, for example, may combine old and new paradigm types of marketing objectives. If there is a substantial fee-for-service segment in the market, the emergency department marketing plan may specify "X" growth in chest pain business from the commercially insured or Medicare or Medicaid market. At the same time, however, it may also specify an objective relating to its managed-care constituents. Recognizing that many people utilize the emergency department inappropriately and therefore use resources unnecessarily, a marketing objective may state, "To reduce the amount of inappropriate utilization of the emergency department on the part of capitated customers." This marketing plan will, in effect, be aimed at de-marketing certain behaviors. It will work to make the market aware of and prefer alternatives to the ED such as calling a nurse line or using an urgent care alternative after hours.

A format for developing healthcare marketing plans that gets results will not only set appropriate and measurable marketing objectives, it will also establish the **worth** of those marketing objectives in terms of incremental revenue. Establishing the worth of the objectives sets up the appropriate dialogue between investment and return. If the marketing plan can secure $500,000 in incremental revenue through increased business, then it is much easier for leadership to make a decision on what it's worth investing to secure a $500,000 incremental revenue gain.

A simple formula for establishing the worth of a marketing objective is, "X" increase in volume times charges less contractual adjustments less the costs of providing the service less the costs of the marketing plan. A typical example of establishing the worth of the marketing objective is the following for an emergency department marketing plan still working in a highly traditional marketplace.

Forty thousand patients were seen in the Emergency Department last year. A 5% increase in visits equates to 2,000 additional visits (5% x 40,000). At $125 per average visit, that equates to an additional $250,000 in charges (2,000 x $125).

15% of Emergency Department visits are admitted. That equates to an additional 300 admissions (15% x 2,000). At an average of

$4,500 per admission, that equates to $1,350,000 in additional charges. Total additional charges therefore = $1,600,000 ($250,000 + $1,350,000).

At an average contractual adjustment rate of 70%, the amount collected is $1,120,000 ($1,600,000 x 70%).

Less the additional expenses for handling the increased business of $200,000 and less the costs of the marketing plan implementation of $150,000 = **incremental revenue** of **$770,000** ($1,120,000 - $350,000).

Establishing the worth of a marketing objective makes tracking progress towards the marketing objective that much more important. By clearly operating within a return on investment format, marketing begins to gain stature in the organization. Marketing can and does generate revenue. It is not additional overhead, it is truly investment.

How does one evaluate marketing in a healthcare organization? That isn't a difficult question to answer for an organization that has set the worth of its key marketing objectives in terms of incremental revenue. Has it reached those objectives or not? If it has, no one has any difficulty in evaluating marketing effectiveness.

As one chief executive officer in a very successful hospital said, "I don't want my board evaluating every single move I make for its impact on the bottom line. I want to be free to orchestrate the whole to achieve the bottom line. As long as I bring in those results, that's what they should be evaluating, not every individual act or step." So it is for a marketing program. It is not an individual ad or radio commercial that will produce the return on investment promised. It is the whole, coordinated marketing program as outlined in a marketing plan that will produce those measurable results.

Hallmark #3: **The format for developing healthcare marketing plans that get results should be simple and memorable.**

A simple and memorable format allows those who go through the process of developing a marketing plan to be able to transfer the skills learned to other settings. It should be simple and memorable, but it should incorporate all the classic steps of effective marketing.

The method for developing the marketing plan should be easy to follow for participants and the marketing team, but at the same time, it should incorporate the best of classic marketing management so that the participants begin to understand the depth of marketing theory and its applicability to their practical situations. Once participants in a marketing team have begun to appreciate marketing, they will take that interest and those skills to their next challenges. Over time, quality marketing management begins to pervade the organization.

When marketing team participants follow a method that incorporates the best of strategic marketing, they will not jump prematurely to strategy and tactics. They will not decide what the marketing plan should address until they've done a careful job of analyzing what the market desires. Even more importantly, the marketing team will not jump to promotion before participants have addressed the other "P"s of the marketing mix.

At the outset, physicians and line managers participating in a marketing team may not understand why they are being asked to be involved. They don't feel they know anything about marketing. They feel that marketing plan development should be the job of the marketing department. They probably think that marketing equates with promotion, sales, and advertising. To them, their roles as clinical professionals and patient care advocates are 180 degrees different from the unseemly, if not unsavory, involvements such as selling and hucksterism. It is only when they have gone step-by-step through a marketing planning process that they begin to understand why they are there and why it is critically important for them to be there. If the marketing planning is successful, they will begin to change their own self-concept. They will begin to think of themselves without apology as "marketers." That will not be a contradiction to their professional roles or to their obligations to first serve patients, that identity will be perceived as an asset. Marketing is indeed the management discipline that breaks the complicated product healthcare is into its component parts, and then puts it back together again for customer satisfaction. It is not anti-thetical to "serving patients," it is the left brain set of skills that frees an organization to make good on its high-sounding intentions. Marketing management skills undergird the turn to the customer.

It was encouraging to the vice-president of marketing at a university hospital, for example, when an eminent professor of surgery commented enthusiastically upon the completion of their marketing plan together, "I never knew there was so much to this marketing. I always thought it was doing brochures and promoting ourselves. I had no idea that there was so much more to it and that it was so satisfying." This professor of surgery had asked the marketing department for help in putting together a marketing plan for a new breast center. The vice-president of marketing turned around and asked him and the key medical oncology, plastic surgery, radiation oncology, and pathology leadership to join in a marketing team and participate in a three-step, two-hour each step, marketing planning process. As a result of their participation, the participants not only could see what they needed to do to shift marketshare, they felt enriched by the exposure to classic marketing. The promotion campaign that was one of the tactics identified in the marketing plan was that much more successful as a result.

It was, of course, more important for that vice-president of marketing to involve these key faculty members in a marketing planning process than it was for him to develop a marketing plan through his own auspices in splendid isolation. He did more for the organization by helping these participants "learn marketing by doing marketing" than he would have by doing it himself.

The method that the Rynne Marketing Group developed years ago and has used and taught for the last dozen years in healthcare is the STRAP method of marketing management and planning. The method has proved helpful for many, flexible in its application, and productive of marketplace results. Individuals and organizations that have learned the STRAP method have been able to use it in many different settings to meet many different types of marketing challenges. It is nothing other than classic marketing put in a simple, easy-to-follow acrostic. It can serve, therefore, as a useful tool for healthcare marketing executives working with nonprofessional marketers within healthcare organizations. Teaching them to follow the STRAP method introduces them to the joys of discovery that come from classic marketing and to the satisfaction that comes from increased impact on the marketplace. Using the method, therefore, continually reinforces to those using it the value of classic marketing.

STRAP stands for:

S	egment the market
T	arget priority segments
R	esearch the priority segments
A	ppraise existing exchange relationships in the light of the market research
P	lay with the 4 "P"s of the marketing mix

USING THE STRAP METHOD OF MARKETING MANAGEMENT AND MARKETING PLAN DEVELOPMENT

Once a marketing team has reviewed the relevant marketing information and conducted its own SWOT analysis, the first step of synthesis is to review and then select the priority target market segments for the marketing plan.

S *egment the Market*

Segmenting the market moves marketing team members away from a "one size fits all" mentality. One service aimed at satisfying everybody most likely will not fully satisfy anybody. In actuality, a given market is broken into multiple segments, each with a slightly different constellation of needs, preferences, and ways of making their decisions. Some segments are more important than others. Some serve in a "channel of decision making" as gurus, influencers, if not gatekeepers for others. By reflecting on the key segments, the marketing team will move away from generic strategies and tactics and begin to see strategies and tactics that will be specifically valuable for reaching particular segments.

Segmentation is discerning the subgroupings in a market which, properly understood and properly addressed, produce marketplace rewards. Segmentation is selecting the aggregates within a market that, if targeted, return the greatest dent for one's marketing dinero (give proportionately greater returns).

Segmentation gives the marketer more useful categories with which to work. By breaking markets into subsets, the marketer has more usable categories for research, for plumbing attitudes, and for gauging likely responses to various marketing strategies. Working with segments, the marketer is better able to match resource investments . . . with predictable outcomes.

Segmentation is a necessary compromise between approaching a market as a whole and approaching each individual within the market. Understanding each individual's separate needs and wants and custom-fashioning a service to individuals one by one would be very effective. It also would probably not be affordable or practical. Segmentation presumes that individuals cluster around common characteristics and needs and provides the marketer some efficiency of resources. As such, it is a halfway measure between addressing customers as anonymous, faceless masses and one by one.

A marketing team may already be quite adept at breaking its generic market into key segments. At the very least, the marketing team will appreciate that a marketing plan will require distinct strategies for referral sources, managed-care companies, and end users, i.e., consumers or patients. But it will be most likely helpful for the healthcare marketing executive to stimulate at the outset more nuanced and imaginative thinking about segments in the market before targeting some over others. Some segments in the market may be much more important than others. Some may not spontaneously come to mind or be appreciated in terms of their importance by members of the marketing team.

The first-cut approaches to segmentation are rather straightforward and it makes sense to first consider those traditional approaches to segmentation, namely:

- Geographic segmentation

- Demographic segmentation

- Lifestyle segmentation

- Place on the decision channel segmentation

Geographic Segmentation

At times, various geographic segments will be target segments in and of themselves: particular cities, counties, communities, neighborhoods, zip codes, subdivisions, or census tracts may be more attractive than others for a given service.

Most often, however, geographic variables are used in combination with other segmentation approaches such as demographic or place on the decision channel variables. At a certain point, the marketer has to tie a segment to a location or an address in order to reach and communicate with the segment. The geographic variable ties in with a demographic variable as in "working class adult males in the collar suburbs," or with decision channel variables as in "urologists in the downtown area," or with lifestyle variables as in "those who exercise strenuously four times a week in these six zip codes," or with any number of meaningful combinations as in "Japanese first time mothers in these three affluent suburbs."

Demographic Segmentation

Demographic segmenting draws on, as appropriate, all the thousands of pieces of information in the United States Census.

For particular markets and for particular services other demographic variables may be predictive, not of utilization, but of preferences in the ways services are delivered. The demographic variables begin to overlay with lifestyle variables.

Reviewing the demographic variables is an important second cut at a given marketplace. Used in combination with other segmentation approaches, demographic segmentation begins to put the marketer closer to some of the underlying dynamics of the marketplace.

Lifestyle Segmentation

Some groups of people have preferred values, attitudes, and stances towards themselves, life, and the future.

At times, lifestyle segments cut across demographic categories. For example, the Corvette owner doesn't fit into any demographic categories, but cuts across age, income, education, and occupation categories. The Corvette owner is understood more clearly in terms of lifestyle—a certain attitude towards life, themselves, and others.

Some lifestyle segmentation variables have been used in healthcare to guide strategy and identify predictors of utilization. Take, for example, the schema describing the breakdown of a given population's attitude toward the purchase of **new products**.

Figure 5-10: Bell Curve of Statistical Distribution

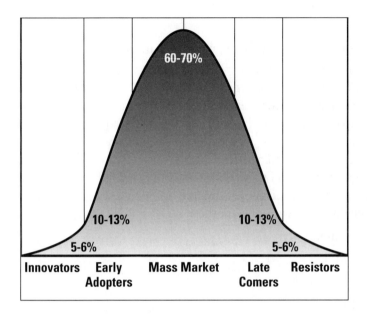

The bell curve of statistical distribution: certain percentages of a given population as innovators, early adopters, the mass market, laggards, and resisters, influence the marketing plan for any *new* healthcare service.

Take for example, healthcare organizations marketing health promotion services to industry.

If they segment companies geographically or demographically such as by size of company or by blue collar or white collar firms, it doesn't correlate with purchase decisions. Larger or smaller, blue collar or white collar status are not variables predictive of purchasing behaviors.

Instead, they should segment companies by their attitudes to the new—a lifestyle variable. Select companies that evidence "innovator" or "early adopter" behaviors vis-à-vis their employees. Sales will be much greater for those who segment this way than those who segment using mere geographic or demographic approaches. Missionary, fruitless sales calls are less frequent. Sales calls are more efficient and productive if salespeople are calling on those who are more ready to respond.

When introducing a new idea such as a PHO to physicians, recognize that the laggards and resisters will embrace the concept slowly. It is virtually impossible to have a whole population embrace a new idea overnight. Start and work with the physicians who are innovators. Acceptance will eventually work its way through the whole population.

Place on the Decision Channel Segmentation

This approach proves valuable in many healthcare situations. It pushes the marketing team to ask who the customer really is. Recognizing that for healthcare services there are frequently other participants in the decision making process than just the end user of the service, it attempts to identify precisely how the decision to utilize a service is made. It recognizes that there is a channel of decision making in the same way that there is a channel of distribution. Participants play various roles in the channel. Are any of the following at work, and how do they interact with one another?

- Prompter
- End user
- Decision maker
- Tiebreaker
- Purse string holder
- Influencer
- Advisor
- Gatekeeper

Take, for example, home care services. Who is the customer? Whom does the home care service need to satisfy? Analysis indicates that the heaviest users of home care services are the chronically ill, the persons over 65 trying to maintain an independent lifestyle. Further analysis indicates that proportionately fewer people hook up with home care services directly from their homes. Most hook up with home care following a hospital stay. Who then is the customer? Not, in this case, the end user, because most of the time the older person's family or loved ones are actively involved in the decision and selection process. Rarely does the older person make the selection in a solitary way. In fact, most of the time the family, usually the daughter or daughter-in-law, has compared alternative home care providers, done some interviewing, and makes the selection.

The decision maker, however, in turn depends on advisers. Family members do not at the outset know much about home care agencies and don't know how to choose one from another. Typically, therefore, they turn to advisors. At times, the advisor is their personal physician.

In turn, physicians depend on discharge planners for ongoing information on and appraisal of home care services vendors. They depend on the staff members, the social workers whose job it is to gather, keep, and assess comparative information on home care agencies as well as nursing homes and other aftercare and supportive services. The discharge planner, it turns out, is the repository of information, comparative assessments, and recommendations on home care services to the entire decision making channel: the patient/end user, the family member/decision maker and the physician/advisor. The discharge planner is the true gatekeeper and critical influence over the whole channel.

A home care marketing team needs to make sure, therefore, that the service is designed and delivered in such a way that it produces satisfaction on the part of discharge planners—above all.

"Lush, Underserved" Segmentation

Beyond geographic, demographic, lifestyle, and place on the decision channel segmentation comes a way of looking at the market which yields great returns. Learning to see the **lush, underserved segments** in a market puts a marketing team in touch with the underlying dynamics in the marketplace and reveals tactics which produce efficient returns. Identifying lush, underserved segments gives a marketer power over a market.

A lush segment has three characteristics:

1) It is sufficiently large to warrant attention.

2) It can pay its way.

3) It is a distinct benefit segment. All things being equal, it chooses one service over another because of a benefit that overrides other decision variables. The benefit sought determines choice and behavior.

If a lush segment is at the same time overlooked or underserved by competitors, by targeting and satisfying the underserved segment better than the competition, one can pick up market share quickly.

For example, for some women in the market for an obstetric service, epidural anesthesia is such a key value that, all other things being equal, it will determine the choice of one provider over another. For another segment, availability of an LDRP option, i.e., labor, delivery, recovery, and postpartum in the same room, is such an important benefit that it will determine the segment's selection of one provider over another. For still another segment, the availability of a vaginal delivery after a C-section will be the determinative decision variable. If one provider offers the option and others do not, the provider that does will pick up the business of that segment and increase market share equivalent to the size of the newly satisfied segment. The provider that offers epidural anesthesia will pick up that segment if others don't offer it.

If competitors don't have LDRP, the provider that offers the LDRP option will pick up the business of that segment. The VBAC (vaginal birth after C-section) segment will go where it can receive satisfaction. Each time a provider identifies and satisfies a lush, underserved segment the provider gains market share.

Satisfying the segment means the segment will *use* you, not be disposed to you, not consider you, not be aware of you, but *use* you, because the benefit sought correlates with choice.

Figure 5-11: Senior Services

Senior Services

Demographic	Geographic	Lifestyle	Lush, Underserved
65 + segment	Seniors in communities less than twenty minutes away	The Go-go; the No-go; the Slow-go 65 + segment	The portion of the 65 + segment that is frustrated with Medicare paperwork and who would switch allegiance if made a better offer

Emergency Room

Demographic	Geographic	Lifestyle	Lush, Underserved
Families with children under 12	People in the primary service area	People whose time is very valuable to them	Families with children under 12 who find a pediatrician in the ER preferable to an ER without one

Occupational Health Services

Demographic	Geographic	Lifestyle	Lush, Underserved
Large Companies	Employees in the downtown area	"Patrone" employees	Employers looking for a way to cut the lostwork time of Worker's Compensation Employees

To identify lush underserved segments, the marketer has to combine secondary and primary research. It is not enough to use existing databases: e.g., demographic or PRISM databases that don't correlate with choice or behavior and that merely tag a segment with external descriptors. Identifying lush, underserved segments requires getting inside the customers and understanding what determines their choices. Such internal mapping of how decisions are made requires primary research.

Consider the healthcare organizations that target the over 65 population using only demographic segmentation or geographic or even lifestyle categories. They end up "doing things" for seniors: geriatric units, geriatric assessments, etc. Those initiatives do not necessarily shift behavior patterns or market share because they do not respond to a felt need. Dissatisfaction with Medicare paperwork, for example, is intensely felt by a substantial segment of the over 65 population. Card membership programs designed precisely to relieve these frustrations have successfully shifted market share in many markets.

A lush, underserved segment approach gets the marketer past conventional ways of looking at a market. For example, a planner using demographic analysis and utilization rate data might conclude that a given market has too many primary-care MDs. A marketer, however, looking at the same geographic and demographic data but who has discovered through primary research that 40 percent of the population is dissatisfied with its physicians and is looking for a better offer, because it is tired of waiting for appointments and not being treated as adults, recognizes that new additional physicians in an apparently over-doctored locale will take over the market—if they satisfy the market on the values of waiting time and adult-to-adult style.

Lush, underserved segment thinking reveals efficient tactics that are tightly connected with changes in marketplace behavior. An emergency room director learned that a sizeable segment of the family with children under 12 market would shift its choice if one ER had a pediatrician on site and others did not. By recruiting pediatricians to his ER, alongside his emergency-trained physicians, he picked up this segment and gained substantial market share.

Lush, underserved segment thinking makes for efficient sales programs. It helps salespeople avoid missionary selling and trains them instead on ready, responsive segments. An occupational health program saved much wasted effort by not falling into the typical traps of segmenting on the basis of size or blue collar/white collar demographic variables. Instead, the sales force targeted self-insured companies with large worker's compensation bills who were frustrated with the lack of case management by their current providers of service. Their visit to sale ratios shot upward.

Lush, underserved thinking also produces communications campaigns that yield multiple returns on their investments. Instead of targeting the chemically dependent person, for instance, a communication campaign targeted the family of the chemically dependent person.

Instead of further dramatizing the *problem* the family faces with the chemically dependent member, the television campaign dramatized a *solution*. It showed family members trained in intervention confronting their chemically dependent loved one to seek help. The campaign filled the unit and kept it filled. Its success was built on identifying a segment that was looking for a practical way to help a loved one over the barrier of self-denial.

Identifying lush, underserved segments sets a marketing team on a path to dramatic increases in business. The best segmentation approaches don't just describe a segment, they identify a group with a definite pattern of purchasing behavior.

Satisfy a benefit segment in a way that is clearly superior to competitors, and that segment will purchase your service rather than your competitor's.

$\boxed{\text{T}}$ *arget Priority Customer Segments*

Once the marketing team has thought about the various segments in the marketplace, the next step in the STRAP method is to target some priority customer segments.

Selecting priority market segments for the marketing plan targeting a few priority segments extends the basic business approach that, in a given period of time, an organization can't tackle everything all at once, but needs to select, prioritize, and marshall resources where they will be most effective. Secondly, ranking segments according to degree of opportunity intensifies and reiterates an ROI, return on investment, orientation. Energy and resources will be invested where they will produce the greatest return.

A marketing team that has carefully reviewed the market opportunity report, completed a SWOT analysis, and identified a range of priority segments will at this point typically not have much problem targeting three or four priority customer segments. If the team needs help in choosing among varied segments, the marketing executive can provide them a decision matrix.

Figure 5-12: Decision Matrix for Selecting Target Segments

Attractive	Penetrable
• Size	• Efficiently Reached
• Profitability	• Minimal Barriers
• Profile Fit	

The criteria for selecting certain segments over others are rather straightforward and fall into two basic evaluative criteria—attractiveness and penetrability.

Under attractiveness, come the issues of:

• Size

It doesn't make sense to target a segment, no matter how lucrative, if it is microscopic.

• Profitability

If it is a sizeable segment, it should also be profitable and it is more attractive to the degree that the preferences of the segment already are being met by the business line.

• Profile Fit

If the profile of needs of the segment is not currently being met, and if the marketing team needs to develop an enriched product before being able to attract a segment, to that degree, it is a less attractive segment. If, on the other hand, there is a fit between what the business line is offering and the desires of the segment, the segment is more attractive.

The variables of penetrability are:

- Efficiently Reached

  If a segment can be identified and contacted with ease, that segment is to that degree, more attractive. If, for example, a few case managers at area insurance companies hold gatekeeping power for rehab services and can be reached through a few direct sales calls, they on this score are a higher priority segment than other segments that might be reached only through expensive advertising campaigns. If there is a distinct mailing list for the segment, the segment may be more efficiently reached than other segments.

- Minimal Barriers

  For some segments, there may be significant barriers in the way of reaching them, either geographic, psychological, or lifestyle barriers. A geographic segment, for example, may seem very close until one realizes that the orientation of that geographic segment makes it turn in the opposite direction from the organization. If a community is oriented for its shopping, cultural needs, and healthcare services to a larger community south of it, and your healthcare organization is north, there is a significant barrier in the way for them turning to you for their healthcare needs. It is not necessarily a geographic obstacle such as a river or a major highway. It is instead a psychological or lifestyle set of barriers.

Once a marketing team has made its decision about priority target segments, it makes sense to articulate a rationale for selecting those target market segments. An emergency department marketing team, for example, selected paramedics and families with children under 12, and they provided the following rationales:

- Paramedics

  Paramedics have a great degree of discretion in this community concerning where the patient is brought for care. Moreover, they are an important word-of-mouth contributor to the community's overall perception of quality. Finally, they have some significant unmet needs that the competition is not satisfying for respect and educational development.

- Young families with children

  The hospital is located in a growth area with many young professionals just starting families. Experience shows that such families plan for emergencies that might effect their children's health and are selective about their choices. By involving them with the emergency department in a satisfactory way, we will introduce them to our hospital and nurture an ongoing relationship with them for all their healthcare needs. Finally, we already have a physical design and a staffing arrangement that will appeal to this target segment.

R esearch the Targeted Segments

This step will be the "open sesame" step for the marketing team. By reviewing carefully the preferences, wants, and needs of each priority segment, the marketing team will have its eyes opened and will begin to see strategies and tactics to influence the marketplace that they will not have seen before entering into the marketing planning process.

Most appropriately at this point, it makes sense to conduct in-depth qualitative market research with each of the priority customer segments. That research may have been done before the session with the marketing team, or it may still need to be done and will delay, in effect, the marketing team's completion of its plan.

In the best of all possible worlds, resources will have been put aside to conduct such market research. It is also appropriate, however, to make such research one of the tactics in the marketing plan and make the decisions on the rest of the strategies based on the existing knowledge base of the marketing team.

If original market research is not conducted at this point, it still makes sense for the team to stretch and try to get inside the heads of the priority customer segments using shorthand methods of market research. A few personal interviews with a representative sample of the priority customer segments is better than nothing. A proven method for getting a marketing team to look at its business line through the eyes of the customer is a "cues to quality" exercise.

Cues to Quality: Secret Code of Successful Marketing

The more adept a manager is at understanding customer cues to quality, the more successful the manager is as a marketer.

Customers have a secret code. As they approach a product or service, they know how to rapidly assess, using a series of cues from the product or service, whether or not it will meet their needs. The more adept a provider of a product or service is in making sure each of the cues that the customer looks for is in place, the more surely the provider will produce in a customer a judgment of satisfaction.

Knowing what the cues are, their sequence, their relative weight, and how they work on the customer is like cracking the secret code of successful marketing. Once a marketer knows the code, he or she can own the market.

To understand the concept of cues to quality, consider first some non-healthcare purchase decisions.

Consider a job interview. The applicant is the seller. The employer is the buyer. Research indicates that the average decision to hire or not to hire is made in less than 60 seconds. The employer makes a "lightning quick" assessment of the candidate using a whole series of cues against an unspoken set of criteria. The rest of a job interview is spent either confirming or unconfirming the rapid-fire decision made within the first seconds of the encounter.

The employer uses observations of glint of the eye, readiness of smile, shake of the hand, cut of the clothes, demeanor, carriage, stance, movement, pitch and resonance of voice, command of language, flow of interaction—and says either "Ah, I think I've got something here" or "Oh my, this is the one I've been waiting for, how do I impress him or her to say yes?" or "Oh no, these next minutes will be a waste of my time, but for the sake of politeness, I will go through the motions."

If the applicant's (seller's) cues match what the employer (buyer) is looking for, the applicant gets the job. If the applicant knew beforehand the criteria the employer was using and could set the right cues in place, the applicant would be managing the exchange for his/her own ends.

Consider the testimony of the purchaser of a Honda automobile who realized, as he was taking it in for its first check-up three months after the purchase, that he had never seen the motor of the automobile.

Reflecting on the moment of purchase, he realized that every other car he had ever bought—even though he knew little about automobile motors—he always made sure the salesman popped up the hood so he could peer in and nod his head sagely, in effect, faking it. He realized that he had not bothered with the charade when buying the Honda because everyone he knew who owned a Honda had told him how well it ran. Before he bought the car, however, he had slammed the door hard. He wanted to make sure it sounded solid and well built. For that judgment, he could trust the testimony of his own ears.

Cues to quality keep customers from feeling overwhelmed. They make complicated situations manageable, so that judgments and choices can be made.

The Concept: Cues to Quality

Cues to quality are the sensible cues of a product or service that the customer uses to determine the presence of features that provide the customer meaningful benefits. In marketing jargon, cues are neither features nor benefits, but the link between the two. Features abide in the product or service. Benefits exist in the experience of the customer who purchases the product or service. Cues are proof points used by the customer in the moments of appraisal. They abide within the purchase decision and the judgment of satisfaction, linking features and benefits. Cues reside both in the product as the sensible manifestation of features and in the experience of the customer as checkpoints verifying the presence of features that promise benefits. If the *benefit* for an employer is an employee who will take initiative and the *feature* of the employee is a take charge attitude, the *cue* in the job interview is the fact that the applicant does not always wait for a question before speaking, but takes some risks and volunteers things before being asked. A firm, fully animated voice is another cue. A leaning forward posture is another. Arms uncrossed, unprotective, and gesturing are others.

If the benefit for a car purchaser is an auto that will not be a bother and the feature of the auto is that it is well made, the cues that indicate the presence of the features and benefits are a solid-sounding slammed door and no rattles when driven.

If the benefit to a patient is feeling well cared for, and the feature of the physician is being attentive to patients as individuals, the cues are the physician's open friendly face, looking the patient in the eye, and addressing the patient by name. Not entering the office lost in the chart, but keeping the chart at one's side, sitting down on the patient's level, and greeting with a handshake before beginning business are other cues.

Customers use cues to evaluate whether or not the product or service passes muster. By controlling the cues, the provider can shape positive judgments into purchase and satisfaction.

The importance of cues to quality is paramount precisely because they abide in the purchase decision moment. Any marketer seeking shifts in market share, or looking to make more money through increased volume, had better squarely focus on the moments when individual purchase decisions are being made, and get them right. All of the attention-getting and image management in the world are for naught if the cues to quality are not managed. Getting the cues to quality right is how the sale is made and the lasting judgment of satisfaction is secured. To make a sale and to produce a satisfied repeat customer, the cues to quality must be managed expertly.

Characteristics of Cues to Quality

#1 The Primacy of the Sensible

Reflecting on cues to quality reveals for marketing **the primacy of the sensible**.

Just as important for marketing purposes as having the feature a customer is looking for, is having the sensible cue that communicates the presence of the feature.

Consider, for example, the woman explaining in a focus group how she chose the nursing home for her mother. She said that she looked at a lot of nursing homes. It was, after all, her mother. Half of the nursing homes she walked into, she immediately walked out of, without giving anyone from the nursing home a chance to make a presentation. The other half she entered, she allowed a representative to tell the nursing homes' story to her. The rest of the focus group members, all of whom had made a similar decision regarding a loved one, immediately knew the variable she was talking about—odor. These people all used the same cue to quality when they shopped for a nursing home. They eliminated half the nursing homes from further consideration on the basis of a simple sensible cue. If they smelled bad, they walked out. The **benefit** they were looking for was care that kept their loved one and their surroundings clean and comfortable. The **cue** that they used to assess the presence of the feature and benefit was the sensible cue, odor.

The nursing homes that controlled the cues to quality survived the first cut of the decision process. The others might argue that they were dismissed peremptorily but to no avail. That is how purchase decisions are made. The cues to quality, not just the underlying reality, have to be in place in order to make a sale and satisfy the customer.

The more complicated the product or service—such as healthcare— the more dependent customers are on their own reading of a foreign situation's cues to quality. They may not be experts, but they have to make a decision. They use and go by their own cues to quality. The testimony of their own senses is the most trustworthy guide they have.

Sensible cues are used to indicate the presence or lack of more complicated sensible realities that we cannot readily detect. The question for marketers is not **how can** the uninitiated make judgments of quality? They do make such judgments. The question is **how do** they make such judgments? The answer: they use their own cues to quality.

#2 Importance of First Impressions

The second characteristic of cues to quality is the importance of first impressions management.

First impressions are typically lasting impressions. During the first moments of an encounter, the potential customer is most alert, seeking information and assessing cues. Typically, the customers hold off making a positive or negative judgment until they have sorted through all the important cues. Once they have completed their appraisal and made their judgment, however, it is very difficult to induce them to re-open the case and reconsider judgments made during first encounters.

Consider a hospital in an urban area on the East Coast. Coming up the stairs into the main entrance of the hospital, one is struck first by the sight of a security guard in uniform, with a gun, behind a desk with a large sign commanding all who enter to first stop, check in with the guard, and secure a pass. The management team responsible for this tableaux was trying to communicate to visitors that they were safe. They succeeded, however, in dramatizing the hospital's safety problem, communicating to all coming up the stairs and reading the sign that they are not safe, and as a matter of fact, that the hospital suspects them.

The same hospital, in its strategy sessions, was trying to figure out ways to attract the suburban market. As long as their first impression communicated fear and suspicion, they were making it difficult for themselves with a segment accustomed to safety and service.

Healthcare organizations improve their chances with customers a number of notches if they simply put in place a positive sequence of first impressions: from parking to lobby to greeting to registration to introduction of the patient to the healthcare professional.

#3 Cues Have Varying Weights of Importance

For efficiency's sake, it makes sense to know which cues are the most important for the customer's decision. Savvy marketers will make sure cues that are most strongly correlated with judgments of choice are in place before working on niceties and nuances.

With the help of objective marketing research and using the tools of regression analysis, the various cues customers use can be assigned weights of importance. Consider, for example, the Emergency Department customer. Regression analysis reveals that of the three moments of the Emergency Room experience, the doctor moment, the nurse moment, and the reception moment, the reception moment is by far more strongly correlated with both satisfaction and dissatisfaction. Of the variables of the reception moment such as—triage, waiting time, handling of the family, waiting area, keeping people informed, etc.—the variable that is by far more strongly correlated both with satisfaction and dissatisfaction is the "keeping people informed" variable. Regression analysis reveals that to produce a judgment of satisfaction in the Emergency Room customer, first attention, above all else, should be given to making sure that when a serious ambulance case arrives, causing delays for the other waiting patients, someone explains what is happening to those waiting patients, and keeps them apprised in an ongoing way. Regression analysis reveals which variables are the niceties and which are at the heart of the purchase and satisfaction decisions.

Understanding customer cues to quality provides managers a direct path into the heart of the customer's decision making. As such, the most important issues for managing choices emerge into clear relief. Cracking the customer's quality code is the royal road to successful marketing.

#4 Cues Tie Marketing to Decision Variables

Reflection on customer cues to quality focuses management's attention on how customers make their decisions. Managing that process effectively is how the organization makes new customers and sends them on their way spreading the satisfied word.

In the short and long run, making a customer is the only way to generate more revenue and shift market share. Riveting the organization's attention on the way customers think and decide is the most efficient path to marketing success.

Instead of wasting resources on merely getting noticed or making a splash, marketing resources are aimed at setting up the right cues to quality and ushering customers along their decision paths.

#5 Cues to Quality Thinking Provides an Easy Way to Introduce Managers to the Practice of Marketing

Managers, with a little prompting, can begin thinking about their customers' cues to quality. Ordinarily, when they begin to reflect on what they are doing from this perspective, they find they are already quite well versed in how their customers think and decide. They are not used to thinking quite in this way; they are more accustomed to reflecting on their own criteria of quality. Clinical managers, especially, have been schooled and trained to produce and deliver a service according to their profession's standards of quality.

As they begin reflecting on their business from the standpoint of the customer cues to quality, they find themselves right in the middle of marketing analysis and strategy. Tactics occur to them that they would not have thought about if they were not looking through the customer's eyes. Through this shortcut way of thinking, they find themselves practicing and appreciating the discipline of marketing.

Consider a group of cardiologists, cardiac surgeons, nurses, and administrators convened by their hospital to serve as a marketing team to develop a marketing plan for the cardiology service of their hospital. When pressed to articulate the cues to quality used by outlying primary-care physician consultants, they came up with a flood of insights. They live every day with the issue. Osmotically, they know the answers, but they had never looked at their practices in quite that way. For example, they discussed very pointedly how important timely, clear, respectful reports about the patients' conditions were to primary-care physicians. During the tactic generating session, they produced a correspondingly valuable set of tactics for enhancing referral relationships.

One cardiologist, for example, suggested installing a WATS line in the surgery area, so that after surgeries they could immediately call in a report to the primary-care physician. Without the aid of the WATS line, they knew that they would slip back into their uneven report-writing practices. With the WATS line, they knew they would call immediately after surgery, communicating to the primary physician not only their competence, but also their special concern for their customer's needs and sensibilities. They all expressed some excitement for the suggestion, and felt appreciative of the insights that they were receiving from the mindset and method of marketing.

A marketing team, for example, developing a marketing plan for an emergency department that had selected the paramedics and young families with children as the priority customer segments, came up with the following articulation of those customers' cues to quality.

Paramedics/EMTs: They evaluate good from mediocre emergency departments using these cues:

- Whether or not they are treated with respect by the other clinical professionals in the emergency department
- Whether or not they receive continuing education opportunities from the emergency department
- Whether the physicians and nurses demonstrate a deep skill level to be able to handle a full range of emergency services
- Whether or not they feel included as part of a team. They are not talked down to, but talked to with respect and appreciation for the job they do
- Whether or not they have easy access to the driveway and entrance to the emergency department
- Whether or not staff is prepared for their arrival
- Whether or not they have to repeat all that they've phoned in once they arrive in person
- Whether or not there is someone on staff who advocates and nurtures relationships with them

- Whether or not they have space for charting and phone calls
- The degree that they are provided with follow-up status reports
- The quality of their interactions with staff members
- Whether or not a lounge or a coffee area is provided for them in common with the emergency department staff

Young Families with Children: Ways that they evaluate one emergency department from another:

- Ease of registration
- Speed of service
- Demonstrated skill level of staff and differentiated levels of skill; for example, pediatricians
- High-tech capabilities
- Gentleness of staff
- Whether or not emergency department staff understand their and their children's need to stay together during treatment
- Whether or not the staff is oriented to children
- Whether or not their physicians recommend that emergency department
- The overall reputation of the hospital
- The waiting area geared to children
- Cost

Using a nominal group technique, a facilitator of a marketing team can relatively quickly surface from the marketing team a whole array of cues to quality that they think the customers use to evaluate them. Introducing those cues to quality into the discussion, much as the discussion of weaknesses during the SWOT analysis, makes it hard to avoid addressing those cues in the strategy development stage of the marketing plan process.

A ppraise Existing Exchange Relationships

Once the market research concerning what the market's looking for has been articulated and/or the cues of quality of customers raised, the marketing team instinctively then perceives gaps between the ideal and the expected, and what is currently provided. That gap analysis points out important strategies and tactics.

A rehab marketing team, for example, indicated that a key cue to quality for discharge planners selecting a rehab program is the speed with which a program gets a patient into its facility—because the discharge planners are under DRG discharge pressure to get patients out of the hospital. In reflecting on that cue to quality in comparison to how they were actually performing, they realized they were taking three days to accept a patient because they were requesting a discharge summary by mail, and after receiving it, completing their financial and clinical screens. They could see the gap between what they were doing and what the customer was expecting. In that moment of insight, they recognized how important it was to reduce their admission and screening time to one day. Having made that change and tuning into the other obvious needs of discharge planners, all by itself, increased occupancy from 75 percent to 85 percent.

$\boxed{\text{P}}$ *lay with the 4 "P"s of the Marketing Mix*

A marketing team that has been put in touch with a live understanding of the desires and preferences of its customers will be able to develop a set of strategies and tactics that are right on target. If the team has done a good job with the STRA steps of the STRAP method, they will ineluctably see the appropriate program enhancements, access improvements, pricing adjustments and promotion components of the marketing mix.

Continuing with the example of the emergency department marketing plan, as the marketing team developed its strategies and tactics, many of them focused squarely on fixing problems identified in the SWOT analysis and enhancing the perceptions of the market through improved cues to quality. An excerpt from the plan illustrates the emphasis on "Product" and "Place" issues.

Target Customer Segment #1: Paramedics/EMTs

Strategy #1—Program Enhancement
- Improve the perception of paramedics/EMTs concerning their place

in the healthcare hierarchy by including them more regularly as part of the healthcare team.

- Have paramedics present some of the material at grand rounds with the rest of the emergency department staff, especially focusing on the pre-hospitalization component of patient care.

  By including paramedics and EMTs in the regular learning situations of the department, the department is treating them as part of the team, respecting their contribution to patient care, and recognizing their thirst for additional knowledge.

- Develop three education programs for paramedic/EMTs that meet continuing education criteria.

- Include paramedics and EMTs in the emergency department celebrations such as the holiday party.

  This further strengthens the message that paramedics/EMTs are valued members of the healthcare team.

- Provide work space and phone access for paramedics/EMTs.

Strategy #2—Service Enhancement

- Set and monitor standards for timely answering of the radio/telemetry unit.

  It's a point of frustration and an expression of disrespect in the eyes of the paramedic that the emergency department doesn't answer the phone calls in a timely way.

- Have the same person who has taken the message over the radio from the paramedics waiting for the ambulance as they arrive 95 percent of the time.

  Another frustration for the paramedics is having to repeat the whole report to a second person when they arrive.

- Designate a particular nurse as liaison to the paramedics/EMTs.

- Post signs for ambulance parking only and enforce restricted parking to other visitors.

- Make the turnaround area for the ambulances larger to facilitate entrance and exit, and add a portecochere over the ED entrance to protect patients and the prehospital providers from inclement weather.

Target Customer Segment #2: Young Families with Children

Strategy #1—Program Enhancement

- Work with local pediatricians and pediatric residents to offer pediatrician coverage in the emergency department evenings, nights, and holidays.

  These young families of professionals indicate their preference for an emergency department staffed with pediatricians.

- Formalize an affiliation with the area children's hospital for smooth transfer arrangements for tertiary care referrals.

  These families indicate that a specific arrangement with subspecialists at the children's hospital will make them have even more confidence in their local emergency department.

- Provide appropriate in-service training to support department staff that will be working specifically with young children, e.g., radiology techs, lab techs, etc.

  An enhanced program for families with young children means staff members that are explicitly tuned into the needs of families with young children.

Strategy #2—Enhancing First Impressions and Access

- Offer "pre-authorization to treat" forms through local schools and day care. Maintain forms on file in the emergency department.

  Parents who feel that they are already known and valued will feel positive about the greeting and the elimination of paperwork in their time of stress.

- Dedicate space in the waiting area to children and maintain appropriate activities and furniture.

- Develop and staff a triage program during peak utilization hours.

In conclusion, a healthcare marketing plan will address product, place, and price issues first. Participants' definitions of "quality" begin to broaden as they experience how the market judges quality. That is the fundamental reason why product and place issues are addressed in a marketing plan. "Operations" issues typically have more to do with improving market share than do promotion tactics.

The marketing plan, finally, devotes a section to marketing communications. The marketing communications section will be shaped and driven by the previous decisions made through the STRAP method. The segments targeted and the issues identified as priorities for those target market segments will determine the types of media used, the size of the investment in promotion, and even the content of the communication messages.

A format for producing marketing plans that get results will review all of the methods of communication from public relations to community relations to advertising to direct response marketing, and select the communication methods and specific media that will bring the message home most efficiently.

Hallmark #4: **The fourth hallmark of a format for developing marketing plans that secure results is *detailed implementation plans* that assign responsibilities, devote adequate resources for each step, and provide a timeline for implementation.**

A successful format for developing marketing plans that get results translates conceptual strategies and tactics into a charter for action. The marketing plan will not get results if it remains a plan. It has to be implemented with gusto and precision to secure results.

To keep the marketing plan from going on the shelf, the strategies and tactics are prioritized, and then specific assignments for implementation are made. A vice-president will be responsible for the overall coordination of the implementation plan. Those assigned to execute particular tactics will be given very specific time frames for executing their portions of the marketing plan.

Assignments of responsibility are either obvious, volunteered, or assigned. The better the work of the marketing team, the more enthusiasm will be generated for implementation.

It was not surprising, for example, to see an obstetrics service marketing team at a midwestern hospital secure impressive marketplace results within twelve months of the marketing plan's implementation—because the head nurses of labor and delivery and the nursery, as well as one key obstetrician, had made the marketing plan totally their own.

One head nurse, for example, took the lead installing a 432-BABY line into the unit, a telephone line for new mothers with questions to the obstetrics nurses that they have come to know. Moreover, she took the lead in organizing a baby fair with the assistance of marketing, and so convinced was she of the value of their brand new LDRP facility, she developed a vendor coupon book as an incentive to women to come and visit the unit. The coupons for discounts on baby products and services from local vendors could be redeemed only if women came to the unit to have them validated.

The other head nurse organized a popular women's health day with the support of the marketing department, featuring Dr. Joyce Brothers as the lead speaker. The nurses worked together to staff an open house for a new obstetrician coming to the medical staff. They, moreover, made sure the hospital's urgent care center and other outreach facilities in the community were well supplied with information for women who might be seeking an obstetrician.

These tactics, among others in the marketing plan, were not only on strategy, they were embraced with enthusiasm by those who could make a real difference day-to-day in the marketplace. With that degree of intelligent, enthusiastic marketing energy, it is no surprise that their deliveries are up 20 percent for the year.

A vice-president of marketing at a Denver hospital had reason to take great pride and delight at a healthcare system board meeting. She had led a set of marketing teams in the development of some priority marketing plans for the system. One of the plans had to do with emergency services. The emergency department medical director had entered into the marketing planning process with gusto. His enthusiasm for following through on the plan was already contagious with the rest of the staff. He appropriated to himself all of the learning that had gone on within the group through the development of the marketing plan. He had begun to use words like segment and focus groups and cues to quality.

He was asked to present the marketing plan for emergency services to the board of directors. It was the final step towards receiving funding approval for the marketing program for the next year, and to set up an annual review process at the board level to track the effectiveness of the marketing plans.

One of the board members stopped the physician shortly after he had begun his presentation and asked a perceptive question, "Doctor, what is the most important variable the marketplace uses in choosing one emergency department over another?"

The doctor paused dramatically and said, "It depends on the segment," and he began to explain quite learnedly and animatedly how paramedics and private physicians and families with children under 12 differ in their ways of judging emergency services and use distinct decision variables evaluating emergency services.

When the physician said, "It depends on the segment," the vice-president of marketing knew that marketing had arrived.

In summary, if the healthcare marketing executive pays careful attention to the process of developing a marketing plan: involving the right actors in a marketing team, committing them to an efficient yet enjoyable use of their time, and walking a marketing team step-by-step through a format that produces a steady stream of insights for them in how to better satisfy their various customer segments, and commits them to aggressive follow-up action, the marketing plans will steadily yield marketplace results.

CHAPTER 6

Service Line Management, Marketing, and Managed Care

INTRODUCTION

It is ironic that each of the industry-wide, popular "discoveries" of the past few years—which some would dismiss as fads—turn out to be distinct and important building blocks, not only for the current competitive posture, but also for the era of managed care. A successful physician relations program, for example, not only makes a hospital more successful in the old paradigm, it prepares the culture for smoother collaborative developments of PHOs and coordinated direct contracting. Through a physician relations program, a hospital learns how to work more smoothly with physicians, to make physicians' needs and mindsets an important touchstone of action, and to work out control issues for mutual benefit. That is exactly the culture that prepares a hospital for the travails and pitfalls involved in developing a true integrated healthcare delivery system.

In a similar way, database marketing has prepared hospitals to segment and communicate with distinct segments in its market in an efficient and orderly way. Targeting distinct lifestyle segments, age segments, segments in the women's market, the newcomers' segment, etc., fosters the realization that distinct markets require distinct appeals and incentives to encourage trial. It gives the organization an ability to move prospective customers from being qualified leads to true prospects to satisfied customers to candidates for cross-selling. It emphasizes the importance of developing lasting relationships with customers. These same capabilities, fostered by database marketing, will serve a health-care organization well in an era of managed-care marketing. Pinpointing the distinct segments in the population most likely to choose one competitive integrated delivery system over another, moving them from trial to active support, and concentrating on building lasting relationships will be valued skills in an era of capitation.

No less valuable, both in the old and new paradigms, will be the successful development of service line management capabilities. In this chapter, we will examine the principles and practice of successful service line management, and then look at ways that service line management will be important for managed-care marketing.

In the industry there is, to be sure, a bell curve of success and failure when it comes to service line management. A certain percentage of the industry has been very successful with service line management. A certain percentage has found fair to middling success with service line management. A certain percentage has abandoned the approach. No reason to make a bell curve normative. We'll look at the places that have been successful to determine the keys to that success. Those that have not been successful may find the reasons for their failures in the following analysis. They may also find an incentive to try again.

When Service Line Management Works and Why

High-performance service line management organizations have seven attributes in common. Leadership at these hospitals have recognized that:

1) A hospital is a bundle of distinct businesses.

2) The marketplace determines the definition of a service line.

3) Anoint incumbent line managers who have grown into the role as service line managers whenever possible.

4) Select high-level candidates for service line leadership of restructured services rather than entry-level candidates.

5) Keep the matrix challenge to the minimum. Service line management is perforce "matrix" in nature, but it is important to minimize the matrix as much as possible.

6) Senior management sees its role as clearing the path for the service line managers.

7) The marketing department is the *mentor* and *vendor* to service line managers.

A Hospital Is a Bundle of Distinct Businesses

From the perspective of the marketplace, a hospital is an umbrella for a bundle of individual businesses. The way people come to a hospital, for the most part, is for distinct needs and problems. No one buys a "medical/surgical bed."

In the past, however, that was the way leadership defined their marketing objective "to fill their medical/surgical beds." Instead, patients come for cancer treatment, emergency services, obstetric services, etc. The distinct lines of business under the umbrella of the hospital correspond to the distinct clinical capabilities of physicians. A small hospital has a few distinct lines of business because it does not have well-developed clinical specialties. A mid-size hospital has numerous lines of business under its umbrella. A major teaching or university hospital has dozens and dozens of business lines under its umbrella.

Not only are there a number of lines of business in a typical hospital, they are all distinct from one another. Potential customers choose, for example, obstetric services using different decision criteria than those who are selecting emergency services. Distinct arrays of customers with distinct decision variables indicate distinct businesses. Even when it is the same physician, as in the case of an obstetrician/gynecologist, there are really two distinct offerings to the public. Women choose where they will have a baby with different decision criteria than the decision criteria they use when choosing a physician and hospital for gynecologic surgery. Consequently, a marketing plan for growing the gynecology service will be quite different in content and tactics from a marketing plan designed to grow an obstetrics service.

With the realization that the hospital is indeed a bundle of distinct businesses, comes the realization that the traditional organizational structure doesn't fit. The traditional organizational structure was designed around functions or professional capabilities. Physical therapists reported to a Director of Physical Therapy. Respiratory therapists reported to Respiratory Therapy. Nurses reported to Nursing. Housekeepers reported to Housekeeping. As a result, no one was really running the distinct businesses under the umbrella of a hospital in a coherent, comprehensive way. Individual managers would have a piece of the business, but no one typically was making sure that it all came together in a way that satisfied the customers. In the cardiac services business line, for example, a cardiac rehab manager managed cardiac rehab; a director of surgery tuned into the needs of the cardiac surgeons; a coronary care nursing director took care of patients during their inpatient stay. But no one was responsible for the entire cardiac service line of business.

Moreover, in the traditional structure, no individual was clearly charged with the responsibility of *growing* the distinct business lines. As a result, by default, where the whole service was not being put together from the ground up in terms of the customers' needs and wants—product, place, price, and promotion—marketing was defined in a minimal way as promotion or advertising. In the absence of a true marketing oriented leader of a particular business, the marketing department was expected, in some magical way, to grow the business through promotion alone.

The traditional organization structure provided services to customers once they were in the hospital. It didn't provide adequate attention to the question of how to bring those patients into the hospital to begin with. It concentrated on operations and gave little attention to business development.

This realization that the major lines of business under the umbrella of the hospital were going untended or under-tended—that not enough hands-on responsibility for making sure the distinct businesses flourished—is the fundamental reason for looking at service line management.

Hospital leaders looked at other businesses that had puzzled through the challenge of growing individual businesses without totally decentralizing the organizational structure and discovered the concept of product line management. In product line management, the person with responsibility for bottom-line results for a distinct business line, for example, a product line manager for Pampers in Proctor & Gamble, is held to those results but not given direct reporting control over all the facets of bringing the product to market. In other words, the product line manager achieved results through gaining the support and cooperation of resources and functions all across the organization. They worked through a "matrix" of reporting relationships.

The organizational structure of a hospital, therefore, needed to shift from being purely functional to a mixed model similar to what other businesses had developed. It wasn't practical for each business line to have complete control over all the functions and resources needed to successfully deliver the healthcare service. It would not make sense to have each business line hire its own decentralized housekeeping, accounting, physical plant, telephone operator cadres, etc. For efficiency's sake, most of the services and functions needed by individual business lines would continue to come out of centralized functional areas. Nonetheless, the head of the distinct business lines would be held accountable for bottom line results. The service line manager in healthcare would, of necessity, manage in a matrix management style.

As time went by, to fit a service organization, the term product line management shifted. Not products, but services, are what are being managed and produced for customers. Product line management was renamed service line management.

In summary, the first hallmark of high performance service line management organizations is the designation of service line managers as responsible for the bottom line of their distinct lines of business. These service line managers are, in effect, **mini-CEOs at the helm of a major line of business.** In that role, they are required to hold and play with all the reins required for running a successful business, but they do not have direct control over all the reporting relationships involved. They need to bring it all together—i.e., referral source relations, service quality, program enhancement, employee satisfaction, resource consumption, clinical quality, managed-care contracting—but they must do it all with and through others who report to other masters.

Service line management pushes responsibility for general management of the business down to the appropriate operating units. It encourages the development of enterprising managers across an organization. It holds up as organizational heroes those managers who can not only run or maintain a business but also can grow a business.

The Marketplace Determines the Definition of a Service Line

High-performance service line management organizations do not design the business lines using *a priori* considerations. Instead, they allow the marketplace to determine which businesses will be provided with service line-type leadership, and what the configuration of the service line will be.

The marketplace determines which service lines will receive service line leadership through the ordinary processes of disciplined strategic planning. The hospital first determines which business lines have the most opportunity for growth and profit, given the organization's strengths, the availability of capital, and the presence or absence of effective competitors. Once those strategic priorities are determined, then service lines are designated. The first principle of all strategy is concentrating resources. Successful service line management doesn't happen where all the business lines willy-nilly are given service line treatment. That typically requires too much organizational change and upheaval. Instead, a few, namely two to four, priority businesses are identified as strategic centers of excellence, and then recieve the service line treatment.

Moreover, the definition of the service line itself is dictated by marketplace perceptions and desires. On the one hand, this makes the organizational development side of service line management easier and, in some cases, it makes it much more challenging. Looking at clinical services through the eyes of the marketplace means that some services require little tinkering with the organizational chart to match them with marketplace desires and dynamics. Other clinical services, however, require a major restructuring of the organizational chart.

Looking at a hospital through the eyes of the market reveals that a typical hospital is, from the standpoint of the organizational chart, already halfway to a service line management structure. The traditional organization structure of a hospital already has a line manager/director over at least half of its major lines of business. Typically, there is in place a director of emergency services, a director of mental health services, a director of obstetrics, a director of rehabilitation services, and a director of ambulatory care. If any of these are selected as strategic priorities for the hospital, there is little need organizationally, in these instances, to substitute a whole new organizational form. The challenge will not be an organizational development one, but one of making sure that the line manager/director has what it takes to function as a mini-CEO of the business. On the other hand, listening to the marketplace desires and needs will lead to major restructuring for some important business lines. The cardiac business line and, even more complicated, the cancer service line, require organization restructuring.

As one listens to consumers evaluate cancer care services at various hospitals, one is struck by the inadequacy of the traditional organizational structure to meet the needs of cancer patients.

People in the general marketplace have heard stories of friends or relatives who, because they first went in the surgeon's door, ended up being "cut;" or because they first went through the medical oncologist's door, were "poisoned;" or who first went through the radiation oncologist's door, and were "burned." In popular parlance, the marketplace will respond to a cancer service that pulls the disciplines together in a coordinated way. The typical organizational structure, however, has mammography, surgical oncology, radiation oncology, medical oncology, and the inpatient oncology unit all reporting to different directors and vice-presidents. As a result, the different functions and pieces of the cancer care service are not managed from a unitary perspective. The various physicians and clinicians involved with this traditional organizational structure are rarely doing multidisciplinary treatment planning. It is not until a service line is reorganized, vis-à-vis the patient, that the service begins to gain competitive advantage.

Moreover, listening to in-depth focus groups of cancer care patients, one is struck by how important, in their eyes, is a marrying of their illness treatment with a wholistic approach to their health.

The cancer care service that is organized to deliver not only quality illness care but nutrition and aids to daily living services will be perceived as a much higher quality service—at least as the consumer defines quality.

In sum, successful service line management organizations let the marketplace define service lines. As a result, the organizational box tinkering, restructuring, and upheaval is kept to a minimum. Organizational restructuring is called for in comparatively few, but nonetheless, important situations.

Anoint Incumbent Line Managers Who Have Grown into the Role as Service Line Managers Whenever Possible

For services that do not need organizational restructuring—such as emergency services, maternity services, mental health services, rehabilitation services, surgical services, etc.—when they have been selected as priorities for development in the strategic plan, it makes sense to consider incumbent line managers as the ones who will be given bottom-line business development responsibilities for the service. They can be designated as the service line managers or directors if they have solid experience and skills in the three distinct areas required to perform as a mini-CEO—i.e., as a general manager of a service. Those three areas are as follows:

Clinical Performance Management

This is the traditional zone of competence for traditional managers of clinical services. They understand how to demand and get excellent clinical performance. They understand the interlocking systems involved with delivering excellent patient care. They are adept at managing the human resources: understand motivations of clinical staff, understand the demands of providing care to the sick, and how to secure resources for the clinical staff so that they feel well supported and cared for themselves.

Financial Management

They have learned how to budget effectively and manage within a budget. They know the difference between fixed and variable costs. They can read a financial statement relating to their services. They want a true picture of their cost structure and appreciate timely information on financial performance. Finally, they are constantly looking for ways to use their resources more productively.

Marketing Management

An effective leader of a clinical service is constantly probing customers, both patients and physicians, to understand how they define quality and how to improve the service to match customer desires and expectations. They are forming in their staff an orientation of service and the ability to anticipate customers' needs. They are insisting that issues of easy access, first impressions management, and final impressions are handled superbly. They are looking for pockets of the market that are going underserved and are constantly looking for additional ways to grow their service. They recognize the importance of image management, and are putting in place the bold moves and fine touches that give them an excellent word-of-mouth reputation in the marketplace.

It is not all that unusual to find incumbent directors or managers of clinical services already prepared to take on bottom-line responsibilities and to fill the role of the mini-CEO/service line director. They are ready for the general management role partially because the healthcare industry has evolved.

In the past, managers of clinical service areas were expected to simply oversee the clinical performance of their areas. However, a number of years ago in most healthcare organizations and/or only recently in some, the line managers have been expected to handle financial management responsibilities. How long ago clinical line managers were asked to handle their budgeting and productivity responsibilities is an indicator of an organization's maturity and an indicator of success in the marketplace.

The amount of the training and development of managers by the chief financial officer is fairly predictive of an organization's successful handling of resources. When budgeting and cost control and productivity management are centralized in the finance department, an organization is typically not as successful as when they have pushed these responsibilities to the department manager level. The best clinical managers take great pride at this point in history in their ability to manage and leverage the resources of their departments.

What has not so clearly been encouraged for traditional line managers, however, is the third component of successful general management, namely marketing management. Nonetheless, the best of such line managers have embraced the business development side of their management challenge. At times, without being asked, they have focused their energies not just on smooth operations or financial management, but have also taken to growing their businesses with gusto.

It is these incumbents that are the prime candidates for being commissioned as service line directors. They already know, in effect, how to not only run, but also grow their businesses effectively. At times, their skills have outstripped what senior management has even consciously requested of them.

Take, for example, the best surgery directors. The director of OR or surgical services is, in a typical hospital, responsible for a very large business indeed. In a typical hospital, surgery revenue accounts for 30 to 40 percent of a hospital's gross revenue. In many communities, the surgery business is a larger business in terms of gross revenue than most other businesses in the community. The choice of the director of surgical services is a very important choice for a hospital. The best of OR directors' performances demonstrate the readiness of an incumbent for service line management designation. The best of the directors of surgery already are handling the threefold challenge of a general manager.

- Clinical management. It goes without saying, that a quality OR will have low infection rates. It will have well-trained nurses supporting individual surgical specialties. Equipment will be well maintained and laid out to the specifications of individual surgeons. Relations with anesthesia and other supportive services such as lab and X-ray will be cordial and seamless. Staff surgical nurses will take great pride in being members of a crack surgical team.

- Financial management. The best directors of surgery will have learned to take pride in the financial statements of the surgery areas, both in terms of contribution to the bottom line and effective use of resources. They will budget effectively, flex staff appropriately, use the operating rooms to maximum efficiency, use financial information and comparative ratios effectively. For example, they will know through their computerized systems exactly how long each surgeon takes for each type of operation performed, and their scheduling will follow from that information. They will know, very specifically, the cause of each delay in the surgical schedule and will be able to feed back to the surgeons when it is that they are responsible for delays and when it is due to other causes.

- Marketing management. The best of directors of surgical services will have taken on the business development role as part and parcel of the challenge of running a bustling, competitive surgery department. They might not have called these tasks marketing or business development, but that is surely what they are. The best of the directors of surgery are, for example:

  - Shifting the share of their surgeons' business in their favor through increasing satisfaction. They recognize that time is money for surgeons and if they want surgeons to do more business in their ORs, they will make sure that the scheduling systems mean no delays or wastes of surgeons' times. Consequently, they will have developed a lively spirit of internal cooperation from other internal customers—such as housekeeping, anesthesia, physician office staff members, nursing, and admitting—that lead to an on-time starting culture in the OR. Establishing a welcoming and supportive environment, they can shift surgeons' preferences and loyalties over time.

    Moreover, they will have put in place some of the fine touches of satisfaction for surgeons. The director of surgery at Saint Joseph's Medical Center in South Bend, for example, made sure that surgeons, as they left the operating room for the day, had patient care papers arranged in their individual preferred order for signing, making it a personalized and efficient experience for them.

- They will take advantage of opportunities for new business through new services. The best of the directors of surgical services will keep their eye out for surgeons ready to develop new skills and thereby attract new market niches.

  For example, when cholecystectomies were first beginning to be performed laparoscopically, enterprising directors of surgery made sure that those surgeons who were open to training in laparoscopic procedures received that training, getting an edge on competitors. When other surgeons felt they were being left behind, the director of Shawnee Mission Medical Center in Kansas City, for example, made sure that all surgeons who were interested received appropriate training facilitated and paid for by the hospital. In such situations, the directors of surgery will make sure that the new equipment is ready for surgeons, at times even before they are ready to use it.

• Spot and woo surgeons who may be underserved or underwelcomed at competitive hospitals. The best surgical directors keep an ongoing "hit list" of surgeons, knowing those who only appear occasionally in their operating room. Rather than treating them as outsiders, they treat them as prospects. They keep very close tabs on indications of dissatisfaction with competitive hospitals and make sure that they out-compete, in terms of service and support, the other hospitals.

If they handle their marketing/business development responsibilities so well instinctively, imagine how well they will perform, if given support to do it reflectively, and the way is cleared for them to concentrate proactively on the business development side of their business.

If, on the other hand, incumbent line managers are not prepared to handle the general management role, senior management is faced with a choice—either help them grow into the role, or make a change. The ability to function and handle all three parts of the business equation—namely volume, resource management, and cost control (volume x price = revenue - costs = profit)—is the key to successful performance.

An enterprising CEO will look over his or her organization and take a mini-CEO sounding. An enterprising CEO will look over the organization to see how many managers at the helm of existing business lines can handle the general management role. That will mean typically how many couple their clinical and financial management skills with an aptitude for business development. If incumbents have taken to the business development side of their responsibilities instinctively or they demonstrate a flair for business development, they should be anointed, rather than supplemented or replaced.

Select High-Level Candidates for Service Line Leadership of Restructured Services Rather than Entry-Level Candidates

All that applies to designating incumbents of services that don't require organizational restructuring applies to candidates for the more complicated service lines requiring restructuring; perhaps more so. Such service line directors of areas such as cardiology, cancer care services, or women's services require the same three sets of management skills: clinical management, financial management, and marketing management skills. In addition, they will be on for handling more complicated matrices. Such a role requires highly developed, experienced management abilities.

The key ingredient in any service line is perhaps the ability to not only handle and satisfy physicians, but to eventually lead them. In these situations, when the service line manager is not a physician, other physicians can dismiss them at first as "suits." To gain their respect, and over time their willingness to follow, takes quite a combination of character traits and skills. The service line manager has to be a combination of strength and service. They have to listen to physicians and respond to them appropriately, while keeping a bigger picture of what's best for the patient and the business line squarely at the center of the discussion. As their suggestions and ideas are proven to work both for the physician and the patient, they eventually begin to get physicians' respect. As they perform their other tasks with obvious skill and thoroughness, they begin to get physicians' respect. As they demonstrate their ability to secure resources from the organization as a whole, they get physicians' respect. As they bring to physicians information about the marketplace, where it's heading, and what it is looking for, and that information proves to be valuable to the physicians, they will gain respect.

It is a very rare entry-level person that can fill out this very demanding role. Why do so many hospitals end up hiring entry-level people for what they call service line responsibilities? The answer is twofold.

1) Some hospitals fear that hiring high-level candidates for service line management responsibilities will lead to an inflation of the payroll. They assume that service line managers will double the number of managers involved with a service. That goes back to the confusion about how many service line managers an organization will need and the "not thinking straight" about the services that already, in an existing traditional organizational chart, match marketplace perceptions. In other words, a director of a rehabilitation service who has all three sets of skills will not need to be supplemented by a service line manager. He or she *is* the service line manager.

It is only the areas that require restructuring where new FTEs are required. When the service line manager performs effectively, the cost benefit analysis of hiring an additional FTE will more than make sense.

2) At times, entry-level service line managers are in effect recruited to *supplement* the skills lacking in the current incumbent. The staff members designated as service line managers are not in effect given bottom-line responsibilities. They end up being assistants to existing managers who usually lack a business development orientation. Such new staff members are expected to do the "marketing." They end up being little more than glorified salespeople or analysts, or whatever the existing department manager structure is lacking. This is a departure from or perversion of service line management potential and requirements.

Many of these problems are avoided if the CEO keeps it simple. What are the three or four most important businesses under the umbrella of the hospital? Let's make sure that we have at the helm of those businesses someone who can function as a mini-CEO, and who has, in particular, the skills and energy required to grow a business. All else follows from this decision.

Service Line Management Is Perforce "Matrix" in Nature, but It Is Important to Minimize the Matrix as Much as Possible

The service line manager will not have direct line reporting relationships over all the functions and departments whose services are needed for the service line to operate effectively. The cardiac service line, for example, will not have its own housekeeping staff, or its own accounting staff, or its own pharmacy staff. Adequate service levels from these functions is secured in a "matrix" fashion, through agreements, conventions, and protocols. Cooperation is gained down, up, and across reporting relationships.

Nonetheless, it doesn't make sense to set "matrix" management up as an end in and of itself. The less the matrix *within* the service line itself, the better the coordination for customer satisfaction and business development.

Take, for example, the clinical service where there is typically the least amount of integration within the service line itself: cancer care.

Typically, the inpatient cancer unit, the radiation therapy service, the outpatient chemotherapy service, the tumor registry, the surgical oncology service, and the mammography service all report to different parts of the organization. Securing multidisciplinary treatment planning—a coordinated approach to tracking outcomes and a central access/inquiry point—and defining which patients in the hospital should be considered cancer patients requires the participation and cooperation of many managers, department directors, physicians, and vice-presidents. Pity the service line manager who has to constantly cross and bridge all these lines of authority.

It makes sense, instead, to put as much of the service line as possible into one coordinated reporting relationship. One very successful cancer service in Ohio, for example, is led by a service line manager with the title, Assistant Vice-President for Cancer Services, who has directly reporting to her the staff who support the five hospital-based oncologists, the radiation therapy program, the cancer care inpatient unit, the tumor registry, the education outreach service, and the continuing medical education program. A large sign identifies all this as the Cancer Care Center—which in many hospitals is the name for the radiation therapy program only. Only the surgical program and the mammography service report to different line managers.

As a result of this organizational integration and her leadership, the patient's experience is organized coherently. Every patient entering the system with a primary diagnosis of cancer receives multidisciplinary treatment planning at the outset of care. The surgeons, medical and radiation oncologists, and residents all put their heads together for the benefit of the patient and determine the best individualized course of treatment—before treatment begins.

Even with matrix minimized, however, effective service line management requires a Service Line Team consisting of the key functions and required for effective delivery of the service. An Emergency Services Service Line, for example, will require at minimum the active participation of the departments of pathology and radiology because of their key role in the delivery of the service in a time sensitive way, as well as admitting and billing because of their first and last impression impact on the customers.

Moreover, to prevent their mere grudging participation, participants will be evaluated specifically on how they helped the service achieve its bottom line objectives—how they followed up on their responsibilities. Such teams need to be specifically *commissioned* for the work by the executive staff.

To make matrix management work positively requires, in addition, that the service line team develop an annual plan that they follow and review regularly. Such a plan clearly designates assignments of responsibilities. Participants are in an accountability loop. Moreover, they will meet regularly to make sure that the assignments of responsibilities are being carried out and to keep one another on track. Without such a plan, service line team meetings end up being vacuous and avoided.

Many of the failures of service line management are due to the lack of a clearly identified and commissioned service line team operating with a plan that has clear assignments of responsibilities, and meets regularly. Without such a team and a plan, the service line manager has to make it up from day to day.

Senior Management Sees Its Role as Clearing the Path for the Service Line Managers

Senior management will clear the path effectively for service line managers in five ways:

1) Senior management will establish a regular system for reviewing progress on the service line business plans. If the organization knows that senior management and, in particular, the chief executive officer is paying attention to the key service lines, staff members across the organization are more likely to take it seriously and give it support. Nothing demonstrates "paying attention" better than regular reviews of progress towards achievement and requiring reports concerning variances from expected achievement and remedial action.

A newly appointed chief executive officer of the Franciscan Health System in Cincinnati made as one of his highest priorities a monthly review of progress towards bottom line objectives of the key service lines. He sat with the chief financial officer to review progress of the service lines on their financially oriented objectives, and sat with the vice-president of marketing to review the other-vice-presidents' and service line managers' progress towards their business development objectives. That organization began to make progress immediately.

2) Senior management makes sure that problems that arise with customers or physicians that can't be resolved by the individual service line manager but require the intervention of someone from senior management are given prompt attention. A regular problem-solving mechanism and reporting of how quickly problems are resolved mechanism is put in place.

3) Service line managers receive adequate resources for achieving their expected returns on investment. The business lines that have been selected because of their marketplace potential should be fed, not bled. In order to achieve expected bottom lines, the budgeting process should make sure that they are given the resources required for achieving those bottom lines. Nothing frustrates service line management effectiveness more quickly than stinting, parsimonious distribution of resources required to grow the business.

4) Senior managers to whom service line managers report are themselves held accountable by the chief executive officer for the service line's bottom lines. When the key members of senior management are part of the accountability loop, instead of being above it, they will work much harder to clear the path for service line management achievement.

5) The senior management team makes sure that the information systems are developed in such a way that the service line managers have in a timely way all the financial, clinical, and marketing information they need to do their jobs.

The Marketing Department Is the Mentor and Vendor to Service Line Managers

Many marketing staffs across the country have not appreciated the opportunity that comes to them with service line management. As aggressive, motivated service line managers take charge of particular clinical services and are given the responsibility for growing their businesses, they immediately look to the marketing department and staff for assistance. That moment can be either very opportunistic for marketing or it can be very destructive to marketing's reputation and standing in an organization. If marketing clings to its prerogatives and jealously protects its marketing turf, then the collaborative potential between service line management and marketing can never flower.

One hospital, for example, in order to protect the turf and the feelings of the marketing vice-president and staff, put into the job description of the service line managers an inherent contradiction. They were clearly assigned responsibility for growing their individual businesses, but they were told that they had responsibility only for *assisting* with the development of marketing strategies. They were put in a rather untenable position—expected to achieve the end result without being able to determine how to get there. It wasn't until this inherent contradiction in the job description was resolved and roles clarified, that the marketing department and service line managers were able to work productively and successfully together.

In brief, the marketing staff's roles vis-à-vis service line managers are **mentor** and **vendor.**

Service line managers who are given the responsibility for developing their individual businesses are hungry for help from marketing. The marketing vice-president who responds to that need by saying, in effect, "I and my staff are the marketers," is the one who will not succeed. The marketing vice-president who sees his or her role as primarily **helping others to be effective marketers** is the one who will contribute to successful service line management. To be a good marketer oneself is an impressive set of skills. To be able to help others to be effective marketers is an even higher order set of skills.

Marketing staff members play their roles as mentors in two ways:

1) By providing ongoing marketing management development; and

2) By providing formats and tools for making the service line manager's job easier and performance more successful.

Mentor Service Line Management by Providing Ongoing Marketing Management Development

Many successful marketing executives in healthcare organizations have initiated formal management development training for service line managers. They begin by bringing in outside professional healthcare marketing consulting talent to provide a formal course in healthcare marketing management. Bringing in someone from the outside highlights the importance of the training and brings a level of expertise that the organization will respect.

The topics covered in such a management development program will be:

- How to set appropriate marketing objectives. Making marketing objectives market-driven rather than finance-driven. When making a splash or managing image is not enough.

- How to construct a marketing plan that generates results. How to develop the plan in a way that excites physicians and gets their participation.

- How to conduct market research that will enlighten staff and physicians and even change behaviors.

- How to implement tracking systems that enable you to gauge and fine tune the effectiveness of your marketing strategies.

- How to inspire staff to high levels of service excellence.

- How to develop a cost-effective marketing communications plan using the full range of public relations, advertising, sales, and community relations tactics.

Such a management development program will be inherently rich and satisfying for service line managers. It will be true adult education because it will be addressing issues that they are facing and the problems they are trying to solve every day. Theory and practice will converge and strike sparks of excitement across the cadre of service line managers. Through such a management development course, the marketing executive and marketing staff members interact in a learning and problem-solving environment with service line managers, and begin to learn to trust and appreciate one another and the impressive gamut of marketing management skills. The wise marketing department continues this kind of training by highlighting in-house staff and their capabilities and providing in a voluntary way ongoing information on more specialized topics and skills.

The following management development program flyer (Exhibit 6-1) was developed by the marketing department of Shawnee Mission Medical Center in Kansas City for service line managers and other interested line managers.

Exhibit 6-1: Shawnee Mission Medical Center's Management Development Series Flyer

---

M&P
Blue Tray Series

Grab a blue tray and join us in the Sunflower Room from noon to 1 p.m. for these fun learning sessions. Each program will include a short presentation by a marketing and planning staff member or an invited guest followed by a group case study to find creative ways to apply these marketing fundamentals to projects at SMMC.

Are You Really Dumb Enough to Buy Crystal Lite?

How packaging a product influences customer behavior
Thursday, July 18

Radio? TV? Billboards?

Demystifying the steps of media buying
Monday, August 19

Just Do a Brochure

A walk through the steps of successful brochure planning
Friday, September 20

You Want to Know What?

How to use research effectively
Thursday, October 17

Man Bites Dog

How to make your story newsworthy
Thursday, November 21

Mentor Service Line Management by Providing Formats and Tools for Making Their Job Easier and Performance More Successful.

The key tools to provide service line managers are: a format and instructions for developing a marketing plan, and a format for addressing particular communications challenges.

Providing a format for developing a marketing plan that helps service line managers not only address the right issues, but discover surprising insights as they develop the plan, enables service line managers to learn marketing by doing it. The marketing staff assists them through the development of a marketing plan. (See Chapter 5 for a recommended format.) By providing service line managers with an effective format and tools for developing a marketing plan, the marketing department not only assures a consistent level of quality across the organization, it puts the lead responsibility for the development of the marketing strategies where it belongs: in the hands of those who are accountable for producing the results.

The marketing staff can facilitate and staff the work of the service line business development team, but they don't take over the responsibility for developing the marketing plan. That responsibility stays with the service line manager.

Marketing staff members, for example, at Cape Coral Hospital clearly understood their role as internal consultants and mentors. They developed a clear brochure describing their services and roles vis-à-vis service line managers and other interested line managers and physicians. They positioned themselves as "chart makers" and pictured a very impressive sailboat on open waters. Their themeline internally was: "Charting a Course with and Through Marketing and Public Relations." (See Exhibit 6-2.)

Cape Coral marketing staff conducted sessions for line managers on how to effectively use their services as described in the brochure. In so doing, they strengthened their mentoring role.

Work Effectively with Service Line Managers by Fostering a *Vendor* Relationship.

Some marketing departments cling unnecessarily to control and power and turf issues. They say things like, "Everybody thinks they're an expert when it comes to writing. We don't pretend to be experts in their jobs. Why do they try to tell us what to do." Such laments, while understandable, are not usually a good sign of a healthy working relationship.

The clearest model for marketing vis-à-vis service line management is: the service line manager is the client. Marketing is the provider of

Exhibit 6-2: Cape Coral Hospital Chart Makers Brochure

Just as you wouldn't take a boat into unfamiliar waters without a chart, you shouldn't even think about launching a new program or service, planning a seminar, staging a special event or writing a brochure, without consulting the Chart Makers in Marketing and Public Relations.

WHAT IS
MARKETING AND PR?

It is the arm of hospital administration charged with the design, implementation and evaluation of an overall marketing program that supports the long and short range goals of the organization as set by the Board of Trustees. Marketing and PR takes the hospital's mission statement and communicates that statement to thevarious publics we serve. To accomplish these tasks, several tools are utilized, including: Research, Advertising, Community Relations, Media Relations, Publication Production, Graphic Design and Special Events. The Marketing and Public Relations program is carefully planned and plotted to keep Cape Coral Hospital on courseat all times.

In addition to corporate program development, Marketing & PR functions as an in-house advertising and public relations firm, offering full support services to hospital departments and to our medical staff.

Marketing & PR is part of the Corporate Development division, along with Physician Services, New Business Development and Wellness Services.

contracted or purchased services. With that model in place, a number of issues will be resolved.

- The ultimate approval authority for a marketing plan, a marketing communications program, and the design of a marketing research study is with the service line manager as the client. The marketing professional, however, has the specialized expertise to manage the ad agency, market research firm, etc., in a way that will enable the best possible product to be brought forward to the service line manager.

- The more knowledgeable about marketing the service line managers become, the more successfully will they be able to use the full, specialized expertise of the marketing department.

- The more knowledgeable they become, the more appreciative they will be of the specialized expertise of the marketing department. Approval authority does not necessarily mean intervening, meddling, and not being appreciative. It will mean just the opposite, as it does in any specialized provider of service to client relationship. Over time, the more the provider of services demonstrates their insights and effectiveness, the more trusting a client becomes.

Reflect on the relationship that a marketing staff has with a good ad agency or a good market research provider. That relationship will give a clue to and illuminate the appropriate relationship between the marketing staff and the service line manager.

When an ad agency is doing an effective, satisfying job for the marketing department, the ad agency will be given free rein and will be asked to take the lead in developing creative ideas and solutions. Taking this kind of lead and responsibility doesn't mean that the marketing staff has given over responsibility for a project to an ad agency. The marketing staff still has the final authority and responsibility for the quality of the product.

In such a situation, the ad agency will be encouraged to present ideas that aren't at first easily acceptable. If they make sense and over time are consistently effective, the marketing executive will learn to trust their recommendations even when they seem counter to his or her intuition. The marketing executive is always free to veto a recommendation and ask the ad agency to come up with other approaches.

The marketing executive trusts their expertise and understands the value of their time, but on the other hand, expects the ad agency to listen, keep him or her informed, and present ideas in a fashion most likely to get his or her enthusiastic endorsement.

This is the same way the marketing staff should work with the service line managers as **vendor to client**. This model promotes effective collaboration between the marketing function and service line management teams.

The marketing executive and staff are not subordinate to service line managers. Instead, they are in a collaborative and expert vendor-to-client relationship.

The following chart summarizes the preceding information in visual form.

Figure 6-1: Successful Service Line Management

	Services That Don't Need Restructuring*	Services That Need Restructuring**
Best Candidates for Service Line Role	Incumbents with a Marketing Flair	Experienced, Marketing-Oriented Clinical Manager
Degree of Organizational Upheaval	Minimal	Major
Matrix Minimizing Initiatives	Commission the Matrix Members	Commission the Matrix Members
Senior Management Reporting Relationship	Traditional Line V.P. Reporting	Report to Senior Executive with Standing and Clout
Relation with Marketing Department	Marketing as Mentor and Vendor	Marketing as Mentor and Vendor
Type of Management Development Required	Marketing Management Education	Marketing Management Education

*Services that match marketplace decision making dynamics: emergency services, rehabilitation services, surgical services, obstetrics services, pediatrics services, mental health services, family practice services. Larger places can also profitably break out orthopedics, urology, ENT, ophthalmology, as distinct business lines. Neurosurgery is better combined with neurology as neurosciences because stroke treatment, balance disorders, back pain, epilepsy, etc., will best be handled in a multidisciplinary way.

**Services that typically need restructuring: Heart, cancer, and neurosciences and women's health.

A women's health services line, depending on what all is included, may or may not require restructuring. If it is no more than a fancier way to talk about old-fashioned obstetrics services, not much reorganizing will be required. If it is a combination OB and women's-oriented education and referral services, not much reorganizing will be required. If it includes under its umbrella a gynecology pavilion, or mammography, or a breast center, or a primary care model women's center, or a mid-life program, or a specialists' center for women, it will require restructuring the traditional organizational chart.

Service Line Management and Managed Care

As an organization moves into the new paradigm, service line management changes drastically. The role takes on additional complexity, and new priorities emerge. Organizations with strong mini-CEOs at the helms of their major lines of business will be well ahead of competitors.

Give More Importance than Ever to True Cost Management

In order for physicians and the hospital to have a margin at the end of a year of a capitated contract, it is important for them to truly reduce costs. The fixed fee they are paid will be more profitable to the degree that they have rinsed out of the system all unnecessary steps and costs. This means the organization has moved far past estimating costs, but has an accurate picture of true costs. It means an organization has moved well beyond the era of discount medicine, i.e., simply reducing charges, and are effectively reducing costs.

To achieve such real cost reductions takes aggressive, competent leadership. Such cost reductions are best handled at the business line level. The service line manager who is well ensconced and respected is in the best position to lead these cost reduction efforts. Unlike previous cost reduction pushes—which were entirely hospital management driven and focused on FTEs per occupied bed and productivity from an existing workforce, etc.—these cost reduction efforts are quite different. At a certain point, a hospital that is lean and mean can't cut costs of care through the traditional management side of the business. Lean and mean begins to verge on lean and sad, if that is the sole focus of cost reduction. In this new era, cost reductions are secured through focusing on the way medical resource decisions are made. That requires a service line manager who is trusted by and can lead an array of physicians.

If, for example, a hospital gets serious about offering a packaged price to the marketplace for its open heart surgery patients, that requires a cooperative focus from not just the cardiac surgeons, but also from the cardiologists, the anesthesiologists, the radiologists, the pathologists, and the emergency room physicians—all working together to study where unnecessary costs exist and how to reduce the costs of providing that care. Otherwise, offering a packaged price that is lower than competitors can lead to financial ruin. In addition, drawing in a disproportionate number of people who are very ill or likely to become ill can yield negative financial results in a capitated environment. A fine line is walked, making the most of the halo power and appeal of a strong clinical service such as heart, and not wanting to attract the "wrong" kind of customers to the integrated healthcare delivery system. Without real cost reduction, reducing price to secure additional volume puts one deeper in the hole.

Leading and facilitating such cost management initiatives requires the following:

- Information systems that give the appropriate data on costs and quality and their relationships to the service line team, including physicians, nurses, and other staff members.

- Strong case management. In order for a patient to be cared for efficiently, the patient is taken through the whole treatment and recovery and rehabilitation process in a seamless way, with no perceived drop in service. The planning of that sequence of care, monitoring that sequence, and making sure that the patient moves through that continuum in a satisfying way is overseen from a service line perspective by the service line manager.

Service Lines Are Defined as System Service Lines Instead of Hospitals'

As the right cluster of hospitals and vertically integrated healthcare delivery points are put together so that an organization can contract effectively with major employers who have employees scattered through a region, the hospital becomes just one hub of a multihospital and vertically integrated healthcare system. Particular clinical services also are managed from a system-wide perspective. The service line manager role and perspective is broadened to be not just for a given hospital, but across a system of care.

A heart service or a cancer service, for example, is no longer defined in terms of where it is housed at a particular hospital, it is defined in terms of the total system's capacity, resources, and costs.

The challenges internally of pulling off such a feat are great. Physicians who had been primarily located at one hospital are asked to develop a system-wide perspective. Defining the service line as a *system* service line implies the following:

- The end of the medical arms race within a system. It doesn't make sense for a system that is trying to offer the most cost-effective set of services to put in duplicative, same level of technology at each of its facilities in a geographically proximate region. One open heart surgery program in a multihospital system of four or five hospitals in the same region is more appropriate than four or five open heart surgery programs.

- Referral relations need to be changed. Physicians that had been comfortable referring to one set of specialists at a given hospital may need to be introduced to and provided information about the quality of another set of specialist physicians.

- Credentialing and continuing medical education are handled across a system at the various facilities.

- Staffing is planned from the standpoint of the multihospital system instead of the individual hospitals.

- As the identity of a strong system grows, it begins to offset the expectations of the public that each hospital will have an entire high-tech array of services. As long as the service is available from the well-recognized system, that will, in the long run, satisfy the marketplace. Concurrently, the brand of the service line needs to shift from being a hospital-sponsored clinical service, to a system-sponsored clinical service. This goes along with and helps the relocation of brand equity from the hospital to the system. The service line manager continues to build the brand equity of the service, but under a new umbrella identity. The clinical services that have strong halo power continue to be important for a system differentiating itself from competitors.

In conclusion, the stronger the service line executive, the more likely will a healthcare system be able to:

- work effectively with teams of physicians relating to a service line to reduce costs;

- shift the brand equity for a particular service from the hospital to the system;

- manage resources and appropriate staffing and technology across a system, rather than by individual operating unit; and

- appropriately manage volume.

INDEX

283

ABOUT THE AUTHOR

Terrence J. Rynne is president of Rynne Marketing Group located in Evanston, IL. His firm is a leading marketing research, strategy, and communications firm that has worked with more than 550 hospitals, large physician groups, and healthcare systems over the last 12 years. He and his firm have won a number of national awards. He was presented with the prestigious Recognition Award from the American Hospital Association for his contributions to the healthcare field. Rynne Marketing has also won numerous "Telly" and "Flashes of Brilliance" awards from national advertising and marketing associations, and recently won both the gold and silver *Healthcare Marketing Report* Advertising Awards for total campaigns for hospitals over 500 beds for Henry Ford Health System and the University of Illinois at Chicago Medical Center.

Mr. Rynne has taught for the American Hospital Association, the American College of Healthcare Executives and numerous state hospital associations. He holds a masters in management degree from Northwestern University with double majors in healthcare administration and marketing.